AF782627

Cellular an

Editor: Sean Wil

Callisto Reference,
118-35 Queens Blvd., Suite 400,
Forest Hills, NY 11375, USA

Visit us on the World Wide Web at:
www.callistoreference.com

© Callisto Reference, 2018

This book contains information obtained from authentic and highly regarded sources. All chapters are published with permission under the Creative Commons Attribution Share Alike License or equivalent. A wide variety of references are listed. Permissions and sources are indicated; for detailed attributions, please refer to the permissions page. Reasonable efforts have been made to publish reliable data and information, but the authors, editors and publisher cannot assume any responsibility for the vailidity of all materials or the consequences of their use.

ISBN: 978-1-64116-004-9 (Hardback)

The publisher's policy is to use permanent paper from mills that operate a sustainable forestry policy. Furthermore, the publisher ensures that the text paper and cover boards used have met acceptable environmental accreditation standards.

Trademark Notice: Registered trademark of products or corporate names are used only for explanation and identification without intent to infringe.

Printed in China.

Cataloging-in-Publication Data

Cellular and molecular immunology / edited by Sean Willard
p. cm.
Includes bibliographical references and index.
ISBN 978-1-64116-004-9
1. Cellular immunity. 2. Molecular immunology. I. Willard, Sean.
QR185.5 .C45 2018
616.079--dc23

Table of Contents

Preface

Immunology is the science of immune systems. Some widely studied aspects of this field include immune deficiency, functioning of the immune system, transplant rejection, etc. The nature of the components of the immune system is mainly cellular. Immunology can be divided into classical immunology, developmental immunology, cancer immunology, theoretical immunology and reproductive immunology. This textbook is a complete source of knowledge on the present status of this important field. For someone with an interest and eye for detail, this book covers the most significant topics in the field of immunology.

To facilitate a deeper understanding of the contents of this book a short introduction of every chapter is written below:

Chapter 1- The cells that fight against invading or harmful microbes inside an organism build an immune system. The defense against these microorganisms can be classified into two categories, i.e. early action or innate immunity and later response or adaptive immunity. This is an introductory chapter which will introduce briefly all the significant aspects of immunology.

Chapter 2- The innate immune system is mainly composed of cytokines, complement system, barriers, scavenger cells, and chemical mediators of inflammation. It is the first line of defense against any microbial invasion. They provide a generic defense against pathogens. All the diverse principles of innate immune system have been carefully analyzed in this section.

Chapter 3- While the innate system is the more primitive defense against infections, the adaptive immune system provides long-lasting immunity. This system creates a memory of response to an attack, which helps in providing an improved response to similar future attacks. The two major constituents of adaptive immune system are antibodies and antigens. The topics discussed in the chapter are of great importance to broaden the existing knowledge on adaptive immune system.

Chapter 4- Cytokines are important for cell signaling. They are proteins that regulate the immune response. A few features of cytokines are that they are secreted in large number by the immune system; they are highly toxic if taken in huge amounts; and they show redundancy. The chapter on cytokines offers an insightful focus, keeping in mind the complex subject matter.

Chapter 5- The immune mechanism, to eradicate foreign substances or toxic microbes, are classified into humoral immunity and cellular immunity. The chapter also focuses on the functioning of participating Th17 cells and CD8+ cytotoxic T lymphocyte, etc. among other related topics. This section discusses the mechanism of immune response in a critical manner providing key analysis to the subject matter.

I owe the completion of this book to the never-ending support of my family, who supported me throughout the project.

Editor

1

Fundamentals of Immunology

The cells that fight against invading or harmful microbes inside an organism build an immune system. The defense against these microorganisms can be classified into two categories, i.e. early action or innate immunity and later response or adaptive immunity. This is an introductory chapter which will introduce briefly all the significant aspects of immunology.

Immune System

The term immunity comes from the Latin word immunitas, means protection from legal prosecution. Immunity refers to protection from disease and other pathogens. The cells and molecules responsible for immunity are called immune system and their efforts in regards to any etiological agent are called immune responses. Normally the immune responses are elicited against the foreign substances but occasionally to the self molecules and are referred as autoimmune responses. Immunology is a branch of life-science which deals with the cellular and molecular events occurring in the body after encounters of micro-organisms and other foreign substances.

The history of immunology is quite old. In ancient China, people often used skin lesions of patients recovered from small pox to cure small pox in young children. The first successful record of vaccination came from the work of Edward Jenner's efficacious vaccination against smallpox. Jenner observed that milkmaid who had recovered from cowpox never showed any symptom of smallpox. Following this observation he inoculated the cowpox pustules into the arm of a young boy who later did not show full progressive smallpox symptoms. Small pox was the first disease that was eradicated worldwide by vaccination.

Recently the science of immunology has grown up by the advent of new molecular biology tools. Our current understanding of the human and animal immune system and its functions has remarkably improved. Advances such as recombinant DNA technology, immunohistochemistry, monoclonal antibody production and x-ray crystallography have changed the immunology to a broader area. The development of techniques to produce transgenic and knockout mice has also played a great role to understand many complex immunological pathways.

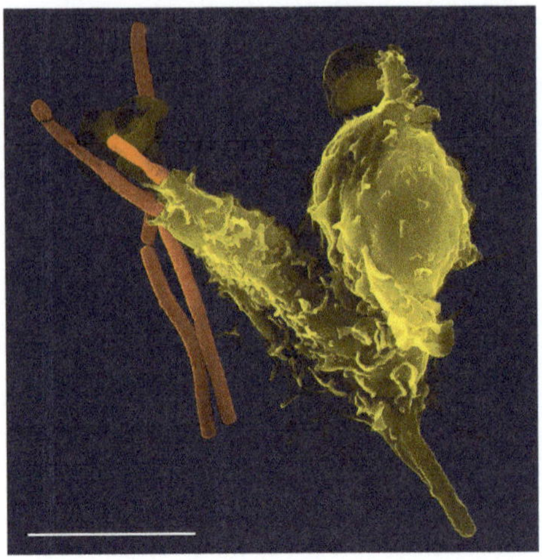

A scanning electron microscope image of a single neutrophil (yellow), engulfing anthrax bacteria (orange)

The immune system is a host defense system comprising many biological structures and processes within an organism that protects against disease. To function properly, an immune system must detect a wide variety of agents, known as pathogens, from viruses to parasitic worms, and distinguish them from the organism's own healthy tissue. In many species, the immune system can be classified into subsystems, such as the innate immune system versus the adaptive immune system, or humoral immunity versus cell-mediated immunity. In humans, the blood–brain barrier, blood–cerebrospinal fluid barrier, and similar fluid–brain barriers separate the peripheral immune system from the neuroimmune system, which protects the brain.

Pathogens can rapidly evolve and adapt, and thereby avoid detection and neutralization by the immune system; however, multiple defense mechanisms have also evolved to recognize and neutralize pathogens. Even simple unicellular organisms such as bacteria possess a rudimentary immune system in the form of enzymes that protect against bacteriophage infections. Other basic immune mechanisms evolved in ancient eukaryotes and remain in their modern descendants, such as plants and invertebrates. These mechanisms include phagocytosis, antimicrobial peptides called defensins, and the complement system. Jawed vertebrates, including humans, have even more sophisticated defense mechanisms, including the ability to adapt over time to recognize specific pathogens more efficiently. Adaptive (or acquired) immunity creates immunological memory after an initial response to a specific pathogen, leading to an enhanced response to subsequent encounters with that same pathogen. This process of acquired immunity is the basis of vaccination.

Disorders of the immune system can result in autoimmune diseases, inflammatory diseases and cancer. Immunodeficiency occurs when the immune system is less active than normal, resulting in recurring and life-threatening infections. In humans, immunodeficiency can either be the result of a genetic disease such as severe combined immunodeficiency, acquired conditions such as HIV/AIDS, or the use of immunosuppressive medication. In contrast, autoimmunity results from a hyperactive immune system attacking normal tissues as if they were foreign organisms. Common autoimmune diseases include Hashimoto's thyroiditis, rheumatoid arthritis, diabetes mellitus type 1, and systemic lupus erythematosus. Immunology covers the study of all aspects of the immune system.

History of Immunology

Immunology is a science that examines the structure and function of the immune system. It originates from medicine and early studies on the causes of immunity to disease. The earliest known reference to immunity was during the plague of Athens in 430 BC. Thucydides noted that people who had recovered from a previous bout of the disease could nurse the sick without contracting the illness a second time. In the 18th century, Pierre-Louis Moreau de Maupertuis made experiments with scorpion venom and observed that certain dogs and mice were immune to this venom. This and other observations of acquired immunity were later exploited by Louis Pasteur in his development of vaccination and his proposed germ theory of disease. Pasteur's theory was in direct opposition to contemporary theories of disease, such as the miasma theory. It was not until Robert Koch's 1891 proofs, for which he was awarded a Nobel Prize in 1905, that microorganisms were confirmed as the cause of infectious disease. Viruses were confirmed as human pathogens in 1901, with the discovery of the yellow fever virus by Walter Reed.

Immunology made a great advance towards the end of the 19th century, through rapid developments, in the study of humoral immunity and cellular immunity. Particularly important was the work of Paul Ehrlich, who proposed the side-chain theory to explain the specificity of the antigen-antibody reaction; his contributions to the understanding of humoral immunity were recognized by the award of a Nobel Prize in 1908, which was jointly awarded to the founder of cellular immunology, Elie Metchnikoff.

Layered Defense

The immune system protects organisms from infection with layered defenses of increasing specificity. In simple terms, physical barriers prevent pathogens such as bacteria and viruses from entering the organism. If a pathogen breaches these barriers, the innate immune system provides an immediate, but non-specific response. Innate immune systems are found in all plants and animals. If pathogens successfully evade the innate response, vertebrates possess a second layer of protection, the adaptive immune system, which is activated by the innate response. Here, the immune system adapts its response during an infection to improve its recognition of the pathogen. This improved response is then retained after the pathogen has been eliminated, in the form of an immunological memory, and allows the adaptive immune system to mount faster and stronger attacks each time this pathogen is encountered.

Components of the immune system	
Innate immune system	Adaptive immune system
Response is non-specific	Pathogen and antigen specific response
Exposure leads to immediate maximal response	Lag time between exposure and maximal response
Cell-mediated and humoral components	Cell-mediated and humoral components
No immunological memory	Exposure leads to immunological memory
Found in nearly all forms of life	Found only in jawed vertebrates

Both innate and adaptive immunity depend on the ability of the immune system to distinguish between self and non-self molecules. In immunology, *self* molecules are those components of an organism's body that can be distinguished from foreign substances by the immune system. Conversely, *non-self* molecules are those recognized as foreign molecules. One class of non-self molecules are called antigens (short for *anti*body *gen*erators) and are defined as substances that bind to specific immune receptors and elicit an immune response.

Innate Immune System

Microorganisms or toxins that successfully enter an organism encounter the cells and mechanisms of the innate immune system. The innate response is usually triggered when microbes are identified by pattern recognition receptors, which recognize components that are conserved among broad groups of microorganisms, or when damaged, injured or stressed cells send out alarm signals, many of which (but not all) are recognized by the same receptors as those that recognize pathogens. Innate immune defenses are non-specific, meaning these systems respond to pathogens in a generic way. This system does not confer long-lasting immunity against a pathogen. The innate immune system is the dominant system of host defense in most organisms.

Surface Barriers

Several barriers protect organisms from infection, including mechanical, chemical, and biological barriers. The waxy cuticle of many leaves, the exoskeleton of insects, the shells and membranes of externally deposited eggs, and skin are examples of mechanical barriers that are the first line of defense against infection. However, as organisms cannot be completely sealed from their environments, other systems act to protect body openings such as the lungs, intestines, and the genitourinary tract. In the lungs, coughing and sneezing mechanically eject pathogens and other irritants from the respiratory tract. The flushing action of tears and urine also mechanically expels pathogens, while mucus secreted by the respiratory and gastrointestinal tract serves to trap and entangle microorganisms.

Chemical barriers also protect against infection. The skin and respiratory tract secrete antimicrobial peptides such as the β-defensins. Enzymes such as lysozyme and phospholipase A2 in saliva, tears, and breast milk are also antibacterials. Vaginal secretions serve as a chemical barrier following menarche, when they become slightly acidic, while semen contains defensins and zinc to kill pathogens. In the stomach, gastric acid and proteases serve as powerful chemical defenses against ingested pathogens.

Within the genitourinary and gastrointestinal tracts, commensal flora serve as biological barriers by competing with pathogenic bacteria for food and space and, in some cases, by changing the conditions in their environment, such as pH or available iron. As a result of the symbiotic relationship between commensals and the immune system, the probability that pathogens will reach sufficient numbers to cause illness is reduced. However, since most antibiotics non-specifically target bacteria and do not affect fungi, oral antibiotics can lead to an "overgrowth" of fungi and cause conditions such as a vaginal candidiasis (a yeast infection). There is good evidence that re-introduction of probiotic flora, such as pure cultures of the lactobacilli normally found in unpasteurized yogurt, helps restore a healthy balance of microbial populations in intestinal infections in children and encouraging preliminary data in studies on bacterial gastroenteritis, inflammatory bowel diseases, urinary tract infection and post-surgical infections.

Inflammation

Inflammation is one of the first responses of the immune system to infection. The symptoms of inflammation are redness, swelling, heat, and pain, which are caused by increased blood flow into tissue. Inflammation is produced by eicosanoids and cytokines, which are released by injured or infected cells. Eicosanoids include prostaglandins that produce fever and the dilation of blood vessels associated with inflammation, and leukotrienes that attract certain white blood cells (leukocytes). Common cytokines include interleukins that are responsible for communication between white blood cells; chemokines that promote chemotaxis; and interferons that have anti-viral effects, such as shutting down protein synthesis in the host cell. Growth factors and cytotoxic factors may also be released. These cytokines and other chemicals recruit immune cells to the site of infection and promote healing of any damaged tissue following the removal of pathogens.

Complement System

The complement system is a biochemical cascade that attacks the surfaces of foreign cells. It contains over 20 different proteins and is named for its ability to "complement" the killing of pathogens by antibodies. Complement is the major humoral component of the innate immune response. Many species have complement systems, including non-mammals like plants, fish, and some invertebrates.

In humans, this response is activated by complement binding to antibodies that have attached to these microbes or the binding of complement proteins to carbohydrates on the surfaces of microbes. This recognition signal triggers a rapid killing response. The speed of the response is a result of signal amplification that occurs following sequential proteolytic activation of complement molecules, which are also proteases. After complement proteins initially bind to the microbe, they activate their protease activity, which in turn activates other complement proteases, and so on. This produces a catalytic cascade that amplifies the initial signal by controlled positive feedback. The cascade results in the production of peptides that attract immune cells, increase vascular permeability, and opsonize (coat) the surface of a pathogen, marking it for destruction. This deposition of complement can also kill cells directly by disrupting their plasma membrane.

Cellular Barriers

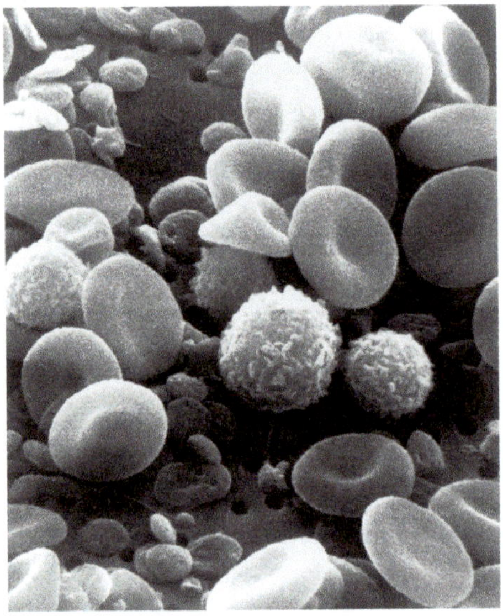

A scanning electron microscope image of normal circulating human blood. One can see red blood cells, several knobby white blood cells including lymphocytes, a monocyte, a neutrophil, and many small disc-shaped platelets.

Leukocytes (white blood cells) act like independent, single-celled organisms and are the second arm of the innate immune system. The innate leukocytes include the phagocytes (macrophages, neutrophils, and dendritic cells), innate lymphoid cells, mast cells, eosinophils, basophils, and natural killer cells. These cells identify and eliminate pathogens, either by attacking larger pathogens through contact or by engulfing and then killing microorganisms. Innate cells are also important mediators in lymphoid organ development and the activation of the adaptive immune system.

Phagocytosis is an important feature of cellular innate immunity performed by cells called 'phagocytes' that engulf, or eat, pathogens or particles. Phagocytes generally patrol the body searching for pathogens, but can be called to specific locations by cytokines. Once a pathogen has been engulfed by a phagocyte, it becomes trapped in an intracellular vesicle called a phagosome, which subsequently fuses with another vesicle called a lysosome to form a phagolysosome. The pathogen is killed by the activity of digestive enzymes or following a respiratory burst that releases free radicals into the phagolysosome. Phagocytosis evolved as a means of acquiring nutrients, but this role was extended in phagocytes to include engulfment of pathogens as a defense mechanism. Phagocytosis probably represents the oldest form of host defense, as phagocytes have been identified in both vertebrate and invertebrate animals.

Neutrophils and macrophages are phagocytes that travel throughout the body in pursuit of invading pathogens. Neutrophils are normally found in the bloodstream and are the most abundant type of phagocyte, normally representing 50% to 60% of the total circulating leukocytes. During the acute phase of inflammation, particularly as a result of bacterial infection, neutrophils migrate toward the site of inflammation in a process called chemotaxis, and are usually the first cells to arrive at the scene of infection. Macrophages are versatile cells that reside within tissues and: (i) produce a wide array of chemicals including enzymes, complement proteins, and cytokines, while they can also (ii) act as scavengers that rid the body of worn-out cells and other debris, and as antigen-presenting cells that activate the adaptive immune system.

Dendritic cells (DC) are phagocytes in tissues that are in contact with the external environment; therefore, they are located mainly in the skin, nose, lungs, stomach, and intestines. They are named for their resemblance to neuronal dendrites, as both have many spine-like projections, but dendritic cells are in no way connected to the nervous system. Dendritic cells serve as a link between the bodily tissues and the innate and adaptive immune systems, as they present antigens to T cells, one of the key cell types of the adaptive immune system.

Mast cells reside in connective tissues and mucous membranes, and regulate the inflammatory response. They are most often associated with allergy and anaphylaxis. Basophils and eosinophils are related to neutrophils. They secrete chemical mediators that are involved in defending against parasites and play a role in allergic reactions, such as asthma. Natural killer (NK cells) cells are leukocytes that attack and destroy tumor cells, or cells that have been infected by viruses.

Natural Killer Cells

Natural killer cells, or NK cells, are lymphocytes and a component of the innate immune system which does not directly attack invading microbes. Rather, NK cells destroy compromised host cells, such as tumor cells or virus-infected cells, recognizing such cells by a condition known as "missing self." This term describes cells with low levels of a cell-surface marker called MHC I (major histocompatibility complex) – a situation that can arise in viral infections of host cells. They were named "natural killer" because of the initial notion that they do not require activation in order to kill cells that are "missing self." For many years it was unclear how NK cells recognize tumor cells and infected cells. It is now known that the MHC makeup on the surface of those cells is altered and the NK cells become activated through recognition of "missing self". Normal body cells are not recognized and attacked by NK cells because they express intact self MHC antigens. Those MHC antigens are recognized by killer cell immunoglobulin receptors (KIR) which essentially put the brakes on NK cells.

Adaptive Immune System

The adaptive immune system evolved in early vertebrates and allows for a stronger immune response as well as immunological memory, where each pathogen is "remembered" by a signature antigen. The adaptive immune response is antigen-specific and requires the recognition of specific "non-self" antigens during a process called antigen presentation. Antigen specificity allows for the generation of responses that are tailored to specific pathogens or pathogen-infected cells. The ability to mount these tailored responses is maintained in the body by "memory cells". Should a pathogen infect the body more than once, these specific memory cells are used to quickly eliminate it.

Lymphocytes

The cells of the adaptive immune system are special types of leukocytes, called lymphocytes. B cells and T cells are the major types of lymphocytes and are derived from hematopoietic stem cells in the bone marrow. B cells are involved in the humoral immune response, whereas T cells are involved in cell-mediated immune response.

Both B cells and T cells carry receptor molecules that recognize specific targets. T cells recognize a "non-self" target, such as a pathogen, only after antigens (small fragments of the pathogen) have been processed and presented in combination with a "self" receptor called a major histocompatibility complex (MHC) molecule. There are two major subtypes of T cells: the killer T cell and the helper T cell. In addition there are regulatory T cells which have a role in modulating immune response. Killer T cells only recognize antigens coupled to Class I MHC molecules, while helper T cells and regulatory T cells only recognize antigens coupled to Class II MHC molecules. These two mechanisms of antigen presentation reflect the different roles of the two types of T cell. A third, minor subtype are the γδ T cells that recognize intact antigens that are not bound to MHC receptors.

In contrast, the B cell antigen-specific receptor is an antibody molecule on the B cell surface, and recognizes whole pathogens without any need for antigen processing. Each lineage of B cell expresses a different antibody, so the complete set of B cell antigen receptors represent all the antibodies that the body can manufacture.

Killer T Cells

Killer T cells are a sub-group of T cells that kill cells that are infected with viruses (and other pathogens), or are otherwise damaged or dysfunctional. As with B cells, each type of T cell recognizes a different antigen. Killer T cells are activated when their T-cell receptor (TCR) binds to this specific antigen in a complex with the MHC Class I receptor of another cell. Recognition of this MHC:antigen complex is aided by a co-receptor on the T cell, called CD8. The T cell then travels throughout the body in search of cells where the MHC I receptors bear this antigen. When an activated T cell contacts such cells, it releases cytotoxins, such as perforin, which form pores in the target cell's plasma membrane, allowing ions, water and toxins to enter. The entry of another toxin called granulysin (a protease) induces the target cell to undergo apoptosis. T cell killing of host cells is particularly important in preventing the replication of viruses. T cell activation is tightly controlled and generally requires a very strong MHC/antigen activation signal, or additional activation signals provided by "helper" T cells (see below).

Helper T Cells

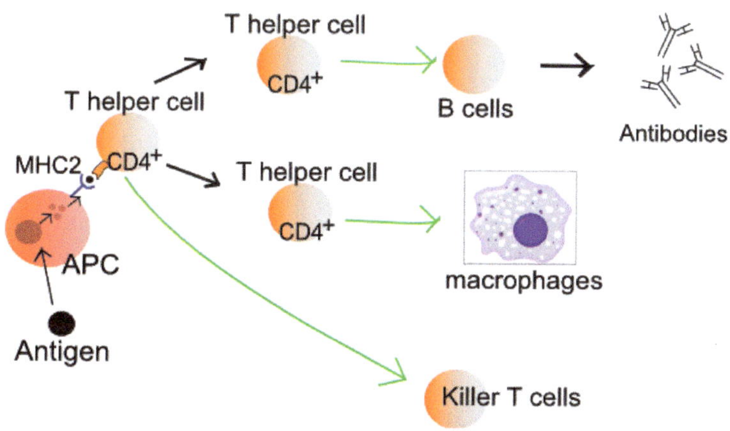

Function of T helper cells: Antigen-presenting cells (APCs) present antigen on their Class II MHC molecules (MHC2). Helper T cells recognize these, with the help of their expression of CD4 co-receptor (CD4+). The activation of a resting helper T cell causes it to release cytokines and other stimulatory signals (green arrows) that stimulate the activity of macrophages, killer T cells and B cells, the latter producing antibodies. The stimulation of B cells and macrophages succeeds a proliferation of T helper cells.

Helper T cells regulate both the innate and adaptive immune responses and help determine which immune responses the body makes to a particular pathogen. These cells have no cytotoxic activity and do not kill infected cells or clear pathogens directly. They instead control the immune response by directing other cells to perform these tasks.

Helper T cells express T cell receptors (TCR) that recognize antigen bound to Class II MHC molecules. The MHC:antigen complex is also recognized by the helper cell's CD4 co-receptor, which recruits molecules inside the T cell (e.g., Lck) that are responsible for the T cell's activation. Helper T cells have a weaker association with the MHC:antigen complex than observed for killer T cells, meaning many receptors (around 200–300) on the helper T cell must be bound by an MHC:antigen in order to activate the helper cell, while killer T cells can be activated by engagement of a single MHC:antigen molecule. Helper T cell activation also requires longer duration of engagement with an antigen-presenting cell. The activation of a resting helper T cell causes it to release cytokines that influence the activity of many cell types. Cytokine signals produced by helper T cells enhance the microbicidal function of macrophages and the activity of killer T cells. In addition, helper T cell activation causes an upregulation of molecules expressed on the T cell's surface, such as CD40 ligand (also called CD154), which provide extra stimulatory signals typically required to activate antibody-producing B cells.

Gamma Delta T Cells

Gamma delta T cells (γδ T cells) possess an alternative T-cell receptor (TCR) as opposed to CD4+ and CD8+ (αβ) T cells and share the characteristics of helper T cells, cytotoxic T cells and NK cells. The conditions that produce responses from γδ T cells are not fully understood. Like other 'unconventional' T cell subsets bearing invariant TCRs, such as CD1d-restricted Natural Killer T cells, γδ T cells straddle the border between innate and adaptive immunity. On one hand, γδ T cells are a component of adaptive immunity as they rearrange TCR genes to produce receptor diversity and can also develop a memory phenotype. On the other hand, the various subsets are also part of the innate immune system, as restricted TCR or NK receptors may be used as pattern recognition receptors. For example, large numbers of human Vγ9/Vδ2 T cells respond within hours to common molecules produced by microbes, and highly restricted Vδ1+ T cells in epithelia respond to stressed epithelial cells.

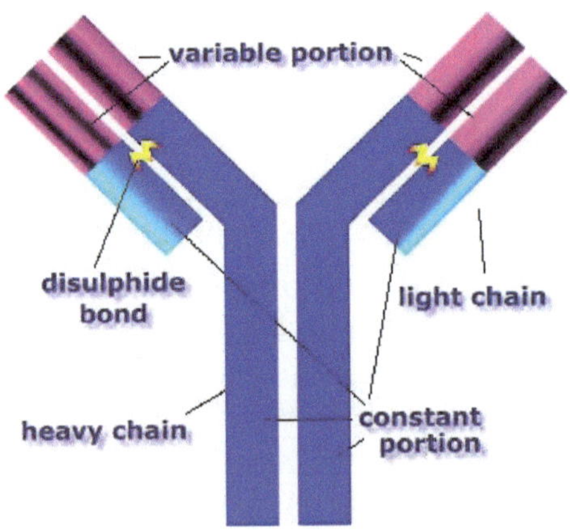

An antibody is made up of two heavy chains and two light chains.
The unique variable region allows an antibody to recognize its matching antigen.

B Lymphocytes and Antibodies

A B cell identifies pathogens when antibodies on its surface bind to a specific foreign antigen. This antigen/antibody complex is taken up by the B cell and processed by proteolysis into peptides. The B cell then displays these antigenic peptides on its surface MHC class II molecules. This combination of MHC and antigen attracts a matching helper T cell, which releases lymphokines and activates the B cell. As the activated B cell then begins to divide, its offspring (plasma cells) secrete millions of copies of the antibody that recognizes this antigen. These antibodies circulate in blood plasma and lymph, bind to pathogens expressing the antigen and mark them for destruction by complement activation or for uptake and destruction by phagocytes. Antibodies can also neutralize challenges directly, by binding to bacterial toxins or by interfering with the receptors that viruses and bacteria use to infect cells.

Alternative Adaptive Immune System

Evolution of the adaptive immune system occurred in an ancestor of the jawed vertebrates. Many of the classical molecules of the adaptive immune system (e.g., immunoglobulins and T-cell receptors) exist only in jawed vertebrates. However, a distinct lymphocyte-derived molecule has been discovered in primitive jawless vertebrates, such as the lamprey and hagfish. These animals possess a large array of molecules called Variable lymphocyte receptors (VLRs) that, like the antigen receptors of jawed vertebrates, are produced from only a small number (one or two) of genes. These molecules are believed to bind pathogenic antigens in a similar way to antibodies, and with the same degree of specificity.

Immunological Memory

When B cells and T cells are activated and begin to replicate, some of their offspring become long-lived memory cells. Throughout the lifetime of an animal, these memory cells remember each specific pathogen encountered and can mount a strong response if the pathogen is detected again. This is "adaptive" because it occurs during the lifetime of an individual as an adaptation to infection with that pathogen and prepares the immune system for future challenges. Immunological memory can be in the form of either passive short-term memory or active long-term memory.

Passive Memory

Newborn infants have no prior exposure to microbes and are particularly vulnerable to infection. Several layers of passive protection are provided by the mother. During pregnancy, a particular type of antibody, called IgG, is transported from mother to baby directly across the placenta, so human babies have high levels of antibodies even at birth, with the same range of antigen specificities as their mother. Breast milk or colostrum also contains antibodies that are transferred to the gut of the infant and protect against bacterial infections until the newborn can synthesize its own antibodies. This is passive immunity because the fetus does not actually make any memory cells or antibodies—it only borrows them. This passive immunity is usually short-term, lasting from a few days up to several months. In medicine, protective passive immunity can also be transferred artificially from one individual to another via antibody-rich serum.

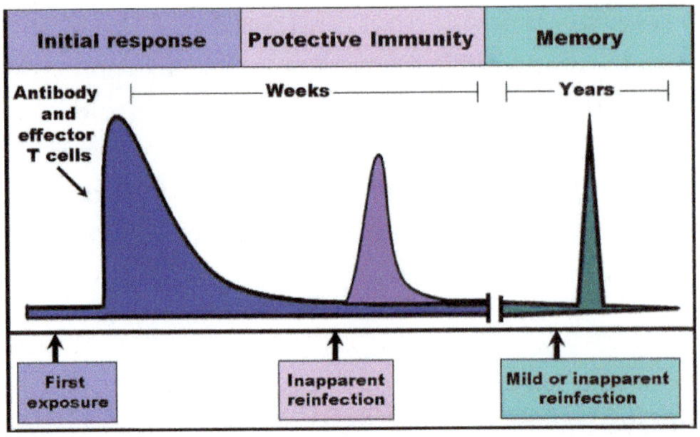

The time-course of an immune response begins with the initial pathogen encounter, (or initial vaccination) and leads to the formation and maintenance of active immunological memory.

Active Memory and Immunization

Long-term *active* memory is acquired following infection by activation of B and T cells. Active immunity can also be generated artificially, through vaccination. The principle behind vaccination (also called immunization) is to introduce an antigen from a pathogen in order to stimulate the immune system and develop specific immunity against that particular pathogen without causing disease associated with that organism. This deliberate induction of an immune response is successful because it exploits the natural specificity of the immune system, as well as its inducibility. With infectious disease remaining one of the leading causes of death in the human population, vaccination represents the most effective manipulation of the immune system mankind has developed.

Most viral vaccines are based on live attenuated viruses, while many bacterial vaccines are based on acellular components of micro-organisms, including harmless toxin components. Since many antigens derived from acellular vaccines do not strongly induce the adaptive response, most bacterial vaccines are provided with additional adjuvants that activate the antigen-presenting cells of the innate immune system and maximize immunogenicity.

Disorders of Human Immunity

The immune system is a remarkably effective structure that incorporates specificity, inducibility and adaptation. Failures of host defense do occur, however, and fall into three broad categories: immunodeficiencies, autoimmunity, and hypersensitivities.

Immunodeficiencies

Immunodeficiencies occur when one or more of the components of the immune system are inactive. The ability of the immune system to respond to pathogens is diminished in both the young and the elderly, with immune responses beginning to decline at around 50 years of age due to immunosenescence. In developed countries, obesity, alcoholism, and drug use are common causes of poor immune function. However, malnutrition is the most common cause of immunodeficiency in developing countries. Diets lacking sufficient protein are associated with impaired cell-mediated immunity, complement activity, phagocyte function, IgA antibody concentrations, and cytokine production. Additionally, the loss of the thymus at an early age through genetic mutation or surgical removal results in severe immunodeficiency and a high susceptibility to infection.

Immunodeficiencies can also be inherited or 'acquired'. Chronic granulomatous disease, where phagocytes have a reduced ability to destroy pathogens, is an example of an inherited, or congenital, immunodeficiency. AIDS and some types of cancer cause acquired immunodeficiency.

Autoimmunity

Overactive immune responses comprise the other end of immune dysfunction, particularly the autoimmune disorders. Here, the immune system fails to properly distinguish between self and non-self, and attacks part of the body. Under normal circumstances, many T cells and antibodies react with "self" peptides. One of the functions of specialized cells (located in the thymus and bone marrow) is to present young lymphocytes with self antigens produced throughout the body and to eliminate those cells that recognize self-antigens, preventing autoimmunity.

Hypersensitivity

Hypersensitivity is an immune response that damages the body's own tissues. They are divided into four classes (Type I – IV) based on the mechanisms involved and the time course of the hypersensitive reaction. Type I hypersensitivity is an immediate or anaphylactic reaction, often associated with allergy. Symptoms can range from mild discomfort to death. Type I hypersensitivity is mediated by IgE, which triggers degranulation of mast cells and basophils when cross-linked by antigen. Type II hypersensitivity occurs when antibodies bind to antigens on the patient's own cells, marking them for destruction. This is also called antibody-dependent (or cytotoxic) hypersensitivity, and is mediated by IgG and IgM antibodies. Immune complexes (aggregations of antigens, complement proteins, and IgG and IgM antibodies) deposited in various tissues trigger Type III hypersensitivity reactions. Type IV hypersensitivity (also known as cell-mediated or *delayed type hypersensitivity*) usually takes between two and three days to develop. Type IV reactions are involved in many autoimmune and infectious diseases, but may also involve *contact dermatitis* (poison ivy). These reactions are mediated by T cells, monocytes, and macrophages.

Other Mechanisms and Evolution

It is likely that a multicomponent, adaptive immune system arose with the first vertebrates, as invertebrates do not generate lymphocytes or an antibody-based humoral response. Many species, however, utilize mechanisms that appear to be precursors of these aspects of vertebrate immunity. Immune systems appear even in the structurally most simple forms of life, with bacteria using a unique defense mechanism, called the restriction modification system to protect themselves from viral pathogens, called bacteriophages. Prokaryotes also possess acquired immunity, through a system that uses CRISPR sequences to retain fragments of the genomes of phage that they have come into contact with in the past, which allows them to block virus replication through a form of RNA interference. Prokaryotes also possess other defense mechanisms. Offensive elements of the immune systems are also present in unicellular eukaryotes, but studies of their roles in defense are few.

Pattern recognition receptors are proteins used by nearly all organisms to identify molecules associated with pathogens. Antimicrobial peptides called defensins are an evolutionarily conserved component of the innate immune response found in all animals and plants, and represent the main form of invertebrate systemic immunity. The complement system and phagocytic cells are also used by most forms of invertebrate life. Ribonucleases and the RNA interference pathway are conserved across all eukaryotes, and are thought to play a role in the immune response to viruses.

Unlike animals, plants lack phagocytic cells, but many plant immune responses involve systemic chemical signals that are sent through a plant. Individual plant cells respond to molecules associated with pathogens known as Pathogen-associated molecular patterns or PAMPs. When a part of a plant becomes infected, the plant produces a localized hypersensitive response, whereby cells at the site of infection undergo rapid apoptosis to prevent the spread of the disease to other parts of the plant. Systemic acquired resistance (SAR) is a type of defensive response used by plants that renders the entire plant resistant to a particular infectious agent. RNA silencing mechanisms are particularly important in this systemic response as they can block virus replication.

Tumor Immunology

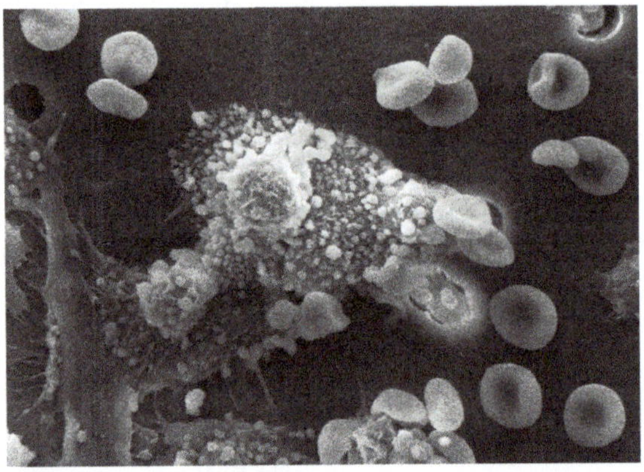

Macrophages have identified a cancer cell (the large, spiky mass). Upon fusing with the cancer cell, the macrophages (smaller white cells) inject toxins that kill the tumor cell. Immunotherapy for the treatment of cancer is an active area of medical research.

Another important role of the immune system is to identify and eliminate tumors. This is called immune surveillance. The *transformed cells* of tumors express antigens that are not found on normal cells. To the immune system, these antigens appear foreign, and their presence causes immune cells to attack the transformed tumor cells. The antigens expressed by tumors have several sources; some are derived from oncogenic viruses like human papillomavirus, which causes cervical cancer, while others are the organism's own proteins that occur at low levels in normal cells but reach high levels in tumor cells. One example is an enzyme called tyrosinase that, when expressed at high levels, transforms certain skin cells (e.g. melanocytes) into tumors called melanomas. A third possible source of tumor antigens are proteins normally important for regulating cell growth and survival, that commonly mutate into cancer inducing molecules called oncogenes.

The main response of the immune system to tumors is to destroy the abnormal cells using killer T cells, sometimes with the assistance of helper T cells. Tumor antigens are presented on MHC class I molecules in a similar way to viral antigens. This allows killer T cells to recognize the tumor cell as abnormal. NK cells also kill tumorous cells in a similar way, especially if the tumor cells have fewer MHC class I molecules on their surface than normal; this is a common phenomenon with tumors. Sometimes antibodies are generated against tumor cells allowing for their destruction by the complement system.

Clearly, some tumors evade the immune system and go on to become cancers. Tumor cells often have a reduced number of MHC class I molecules on their surface, thus avoiding detection by killer T cells. Some tumor cells also release products that inhibit the immune response; for example by secreting the cytokine TGF-β, which suppresses the activity of macrophages and lymphocytes. In addition, immunological tolerance may develop against tumor antigens, so the immune system no longer attacks the tumor cells.

Paradoxically, macrophages can promote tumor growth when tumor cells send out cytokines that attract macrophages, which then generate cytokines and growth factors that nurture tumor development. In addition, a combination of hypoxia in the tumor and a cytokine produced by macrophages induces tumor cells to decrease production of a protein that blocks metastasis and thereby assists spread of cancer cells.

Physiological Regulation

The immune system is involved in many aspects of physiological regulation in the body. The immune system interacts intimately with other systems, such as the endocrine and the nervous systems. The immune system also plays a crucial role in embryogenesis (development of the embryo), as well as in tissue repair and regeneration.

Hormones

Hormones can act as immunomodulators, altering the sensitivity of the immune system. For example, female sex hormones are known immunostimulators of both adaptive and innate immune responses. Some autoimmune diseases such as lupus erythematosus strike women preferentially, and their onset often coincides with puberty. By contrast, male sex hormones such as testosterone seem to be immunosuppressive. Other hormones appear to regulate the immune system as well, most notably prolactin, growth hormone and vitamin D.

Vitamin D

When a T-cell encounters a foreign pathogen, it extends a vitamin D receptor. This is essentially a signaling device that allows the T-cell to bind to the active form of vitamin D, the steroid hormone calcitriol. T-cells have a symbiotic relationship with vitamin D. Not only does the T-cell extend a vitamin D receptor, in essence asking to bind to the steroid hormone version of vitamin D, calcitriol, but the T-cell expresses the gene CYP27B1, which is the gene responsible for converting the pre-hormone version of vitamin D, calcidiol into the steroid hormone version, calcitriol. Only after binding to calcitriol can T-cells perform their intended function. Other immune system cells that are known to express CYP27B1 and thus activate vitamin D calcidiol, are dendritic cells, keratinocytes and macrophages.

It is conjectured that a progressive decline in hormone levels with age is partially responsible for weakened immune responses in aging individuals. Conversely, some hormones are regulated by the immune system, notably thyroid hormone activity. The age-related decline in immune function is also related to decreasing vitamin D levels in the elderly. As people age, two things happen that negatively affect their vitamin D levels. First, they stay indoors more due to decreased activity levels. This means that they get less sun and therefore produce less cholecalciferol via UVB radiation. Second, as a person ages the skin becomes less adept at producing vitamin D.

Sleep and Rest

The immune system is affected by sleep and rest, and sleep deprivation is detrimental to immune function. Complex feedback loops involving cytokines, such as interleukin-1 and tumor necrosis factor-α produced in response to infection, appear to also play a role in the regulation of non-rapid eye movement (REM) sleep. Thus the immune response to infection may result in changes to the sleep cycle, including an increase in slow-wave sleep relative to REM sleep.

When suffering from sleep deprivation, active immunizations may have a diminished effect and may result in lower antibody production, and a lower immune response, than would be noted in a well-rested individual. Additionally, proteins such as NFIL3, which have been shown to be closely intertwined with both T-cell differentiation and our circadian rhythms, can be affected through the disturbance of natural light and dark cycles through instances of sleep deprivation, shift work, etc. As a result, these disruptions can lead to an increase in chronic conditions such as heart disease, chronic pain, and asthma.

In addition to the negative consequences of sleep deprivation, sleep and the intertwined circadian system have been shown to have strong regulatory effects on immunological functions affecting both the innate and the adaptive immunity. First, during the early slow-wave-sleep stage, a sudden drop in blood levels of cortisol, epinephrine, and norepinephrine induce increased blood levels of the hormones leptin, pituitary growth hormone, and prolactin. These signals induce a pro-inflammatory state through the production of the pro-inflammatory cytokines interleukin-1, interleukin-12, TNF-alpha and IFN-gamma. These cytokines then stimulate immune functions such as immune cells activation, proliferation, and differentiation. It is during this time that undifferentiated, or less differentiated, like naïve and central memory T cells, peak (i.e. during a time of a slowly evolving adaptive immune response). In addition to these effects, the milieu of hormones produced at this time (leptin, pituitary growth hormone, and prolactin) support the interactions between APCs and T-cells, a shift of the T_h1/T_h2 cytokine balance towards one that supports T_h1, an increase in overall T_h cell proliferation, and naïve T cell migration to lymph nodes. This milieu is also thought to support the formation of long-lasting immune memory through the initiation of Th1 immune responses.

In contrast, during wake periods differentiated effector cells, such as cytotoxic natural killer cells and CTLs (cytotoxic T lymphocytes), peak in order to elicit an effective response against any intruding pathogens. As well during awake active times, anti-inflammatory molecules, such as cortisol and catecholamines, peak. There are two theories as to why the pro-inflammatory state is reserved for sleep time. First, inflammation would cause serious cognitive and physical impairments if it were to occur during wake times. Second, inflammation may occur during sleep times due to the presence of melatonin. Inflammation causes a great deal of oxidative stress and the presence of melatonin during sleep times could actively counteract free radical production during this time.

Nutrition and Diet

Overnutrition is associated with diseases such as diabetes and obesity, which are known to affect immune function. More moderate malnutrition, as well as certain specific trace mineral and nutrient deficiencies, can also compromise the immune response.

Foods rich in certain fatty acids may foster a healthy immune system. Likewise, fetal undernourishment can cause a lifelong impairment of the immune system.

Repair and Regeneration

The immune system, particularly the innate component, plays a decisive role in tissue repair after an insult. Key actors include macrophages and neutrophils, but other cellular actors, including γδ T cells, innate lymphoid cells (ILCs), and regulatory T cells (Tregs), are also important. The plasticity of immune cells and the balance between pro-inflammatory and anti-inflammatory signals are crucial aspects of efficient tissue repair. Immune components and pathways are involved in regeneration as well, for example in amphibians. According to one hypothesis, organisms that can regenerate could be less immunocompetent than organisms that cannot regenerate.

Manipulation in Medicine

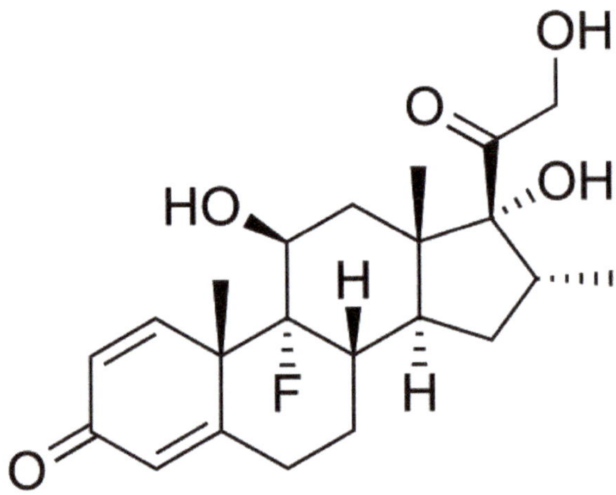

The immunosuppressive drug dexamethasone

The immune response can be manipulated to suppress unwanted responses resulting from autoimmunity, allergy, and transplant rejection, and to stimulate protective responses against pathogens that largely elude the immune system or cancer.

Immunosuppression

Immunosuppressive drugs are used to control autoimmune disorders or inflammation when excessive tissue damage occurs, and to prevent transplant rejection after an organ transplant.

Anti-inflammatory drugs are often used to control the effects of inflammation. Glucocorticoids are the most powerful of these drugs; however, these drugs can have many undesirable side effects, such as central obesity, hyperglycemia, osteoporosis, and their use must be tightly controlled. Lower doses of anti-inflammatory drugs are often used in conjunction with cytotoxic or immunosuppressive drugs such as methotrexate or azathioprine. Cytotoxic drugs inhibit the immune response by killing dividing cells such as activated T cells. However, the killing is indiscriminate and other constantly dividing cells and their organs are affected, which causes toxic side effects. Immunosuppressive drugs such as cyclosporin prevent T cells from responding to signals correctly by inhibiting signal transduction pathways.

Immunostimulation

Cancer immunotherapy covers the medical ways to stimulate the immune system to attack cancer tumours.

Theoretical Approaches to the Immune System

Immunology is strongly experimental in everyday practice but is also characterized by an ongoing theoretical attitude. Many theories have been suggested in immunology from the end of the nineteenth century up to the present time. The end of the 19th century and the beginning of the 20th century saw a battle between "cellular" and "humoral" theories of immunity. According to the cellular theory of immunity, represented in particular by Elie Metchnikoff, it was cells – more precisely, phagocytes – that were responsible for immune responses. In contrast, the humoral theory of immunity, held, among others, by Robert Koch and Emil von Behring, stated that the active immune agents were soluble components (molecules) found in the organism's "humors" rather than its cells.

In the mid-1950s, Frank Burnet, inspired by a suggestion made by Niels Jerne, formulated the clonal selection theory (CST) of immunity. On the basis of CST, Burnet developed a theory of how an immune response is triggered according to the self/nonself distinction: "self" constituents (constituents of the body) do not trigger destructive immune responses, while "nonself" entities (pathogens, an allograft) trigger a destructive immune response. The theory was later modified to reflect new discoveries regarding histocompatibility or the complex "two-signal" activation of T cells. The self/nonself theory of immunity and the self/nonself vocabulary have been criticized, but remain very influential.

More recently, several theoretical frameworks have been suggested in immunology, including "autopoietic" views, "cognitive immune" views, the "danger model" (or "danger theory"), and the "discontinuity" theory. The danger model, suggested by Polly Matzinger and colleagues, has been very influential, arousing many comments and discussions.

Predicting Immunogenicity

Larger drugs (>500 Da) can provoke a neutralizing immune response, particularly if the drugs are administered repeatedly, or in larger doses. This limits the effectiveness of drugs based on larger peptides and proteins (which are typically larger than 6000

Da). In some cases, the drug itself is not immunogenic, but may be co-administered with an immunogenic compound, as is sometimes the case for Taxol. Computational methods have been developed to predict the immunogenicity of peptides and proteins, which are particularly useful in designing therapeutic antibodies, assessing likely virulence of mutations in viral coat particles, and validation of proposed peptide-based drug treatments. Early techniques relied mainly on the observation that hydrophilic amino acids are overrepresented in epitope regions than hydrophobic amino acids; however, more recent developments rely on machine learning techniques using databases of existing known epitopes, usually on well-studied virus proteins, as a training set. A publicly accessible database has been established for the cataloguing of epitopes from pathogens known to be recognizable by B cells. The emerging field of bioinformatics-based studies of immunogenicity is referred to as *immunoinformatics*. Immunoproteomics is the study of large sets of proteins (proteomics) involved in the immune response.

Manipulation by Pathogens

The success of any pathogen depends on its ability to elude host immune responses. Therefore, pathogens evolved several methods that allow them to successfully infect a host, while evading detection or destruction by the immune system. Bacteria often overcome physical barriers by secreting enzymes that digest the barrier, for example, by using a type II secretion system. Alternatively, using a type III secretion system, they may insert a hollow tube into the host cell, providing a direct route for proteins to move from the pathogen to the host. These proteins are often used to shut down host defenses.

An evasion strategy used by several pathogens to avoid the innate immune system is to hide within the cells of their host (also called intracellular pathogenesis). Here, a pathogen spends most of its life-cycle inside host cells, where it is shielded from direct contact with immune cells, antibodies and complement. Some examples of intracellular pathogens include viruses, the food poisoning bacterium *Salmonella* and the eukaryotic parasites that cause malaria (*Plasmodium falciparum*) and leishmaniasis (*Leishmania spp.*). Other bacteria, such as *Mycobacterium tuberculosis*, live inside a protective capsule that prevents lysis by complement. Many pathogens secrete compounds that diminish or misdirect the host's immune response. Some bacteria form biofilms to protect themselves from the cells and proteins of the immune system. Such biofilms are present in many successful infections, e.g., the chronic *Pseudomonas aeruginosa* and *Burkholderia cenocepacia* infections characteristic of cystic fibrosis. Other bacteria generate surface proteins that bind to antibodies, rendering them ineffective; examples include *Streptococcus* (protein G), *Staphylococcus aureus* (protein A), and *Peptostreptococcus magnus* (protein L).

The mechanisms used to evade the adaptive immune system are more complicated.

The simplest approach is to rapidly change non-essential epitopes (amino acids and/or sugars) on the surface of the pathogen, while keeping essential epitopes concealed. This is called antigenic variation. An example is HIV, which mutates rapidly, so the proteins on its viral envelope that are essential for entry into its host target cell are constantly changing. These frequent changes in antigens may explain the failures of vaccines directed at this virus. The parasite *Trypanosoma brucei* uses a similar strategy, constantly switching one type of surface protein for another, allowing it to stay one step ahead of the antibody response. Masking antigens with host molecules is another common strategy for avoiding detection by the immune system. In HIV, the envelope that covers the virion is formed from the outermost membrane of the host cell; such "self-cloaked" viruses make it difficult for the immune system to identify them as "non-self" structures.

Cells of the Immune System

Cells of the immune system are present as circulating cells in the blood and lymph. They are distributed to almost every organ and tissue of the animal body. Their distributions upon exposure to an external agent or pathogens are utmost important in the generation of effective immune response. At beginning, the immune system must respond to the entering pathogen followed by an adaptive immune response by specific lymphocyte. Finally, the cells of adaptive immune response destroy the pathogens by the effector cells.

Followings are the major cells of immune system

1. Macrophages and Phagocytes - They are present in virtually every tissue and organ of the body and respond instantaneously to the entering pathogens. The job of phagocytic cells involves recruitment of cells at the site of infection, ingestion, and destruction of the pathogens.

2. Neutrophils- These are the granulocytes present in the blood stream and are the first line of the defense in the body. They are the most abundant cells present in the blood stream. They are about 12-15 μm in diameter with projection on their surface. The nucleus of neutrophils contains 3-5 lobes (polymorphonuclear cells). The cytoplasm of the neutrophils contains the granules that are filled with enzymes like lysozyme, collagenase, and elastase. They are stained with neutral dyes and produced in the bone marrow. The production of neutrophils is stimulated by granulocyte colony stimulating factors (G-CSF). On an average about 10 11 cells/day are produced in a normal human individual. Usually neutrophils are recruited at the site of infection immediately following the invasion of the foreign substance, if not they undergo apoptosis and get cleared from the circulation. The other two granulocytes present in the blood are basophils and eosinophils which are stained by basic (hematoxylin) and acidic (eosin) dye, respectively.

3. Mononuclear phagocytes - They play a central role in the innate and adaptive

immune system. They are formed by precursor hematopoietic cells and are called monocytes. They are about 10-15 μm in diameter and have bean shaped nuclei. Once enter into the circulation they are called macrophages. The major function of macrophage includes following

1) To ingest and kill the microbes.
2) To ingest and clear dead cells and unused cells.
3) They secrete cytokines upon activation.
4) They serve as antigen presenting cells to display the antigens to the T lymphocyte.
5) They also help in angiogenesis (formation of blood vessels).

4. Mast cells- These are derived from bone marrow cells and contain histamine and other chemical mediators of allergic diseases. Mast cells express the receptors for IgE and IgG antibodies. They also provides defense against helminth infection.

5. Basophils- They are structurally and functionally similar to mast cells and mediate allergic conditions. The granules of basophils contain acidic proteins which bind to basic dyes (hematoxylin)

6. Eosinophils- They are granulocytes present in the blood and contains the enzyme required to damage the cell wall of the parasite. The granules of the eosinophils contain the basic proteins which bind to acidic dye (eosin).

7. Dendritic cells - They are the specialized antigen presenting cells which captures the microbes and microbial antigens, and transport them to lymphoid tissues to be recognized by lymphocytes. They activate the naive T cells and form a bridge between innate and adaptive immune response. They are widely distributed into many organs and epithelial surface. Plasmacytoid dendritic cells are the subpopulation of dendritic cells involved in the recognition of the virus infected cells.

8. Naïve lymphocytes - The lymphocytes that are not previously encountered with antigens are called as Naïve lymphocytes. They trigger the adaptive immune response after encountering with the antigen.

9. Lymphocytes - These are the cells of the adaptive immune system. There are two subsets of the lymphocytes.

   a) B lymphocyte- Involved in the production of the antibodies (bursa of Fabricius derived lymphocyte). The two major subsets of the B lymphocytes are follicular B cells and marginal B cells.

b) T lymphocyte- Involved in the production of cellular immune response (Thymus derived lymphocyte). The two major subsets of the T lymphocytes are CD4+ and CD8+ cells.

10. Effector and memory lymphocytes - They circulate through the normal blood stream and are responsible for systemic immunity against a particular pathogen. The memory cells are important for providing protection against second exposure of the antigens. They are produced in the body during their first encounter with the antigen and expand following their repeated exposure.

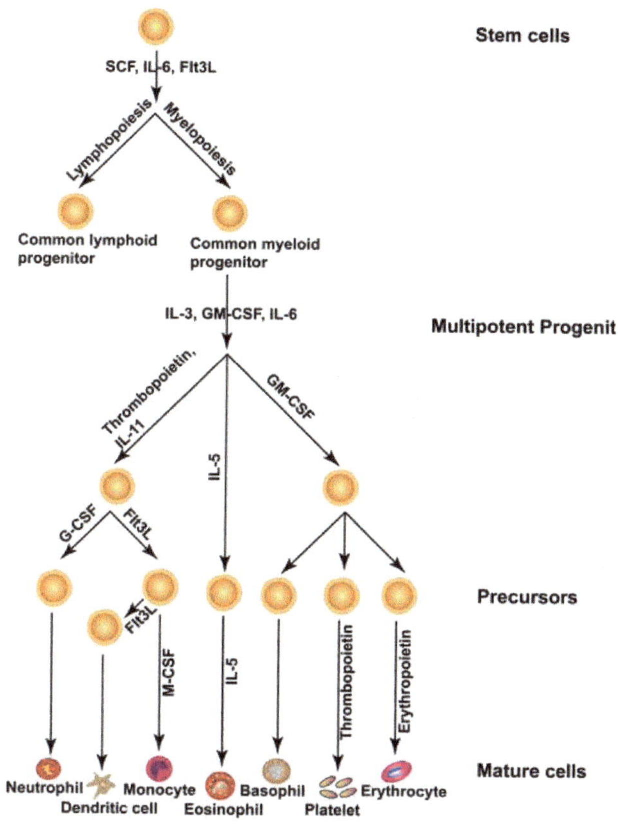

Overview of hematopoiesis:

Anatomy of Lymphoid Tissues and Organs

In order to properly activate the immune system following antigen-antibody interaction, the immune cells need to be localized to a specific area where they properly express the receptors for Ag recognition and attain maturity. Bone marrow and thymus are the central or primary lymphoid organs which produce B and T lymphocytes, respectively. B and T lymphocytes are produced in the primary lymphoid organs and complete its functional maturation in the peripheral or secondary lymphoid organs such as spleen and lymph node . Two important functions shared by the primary lymphoid organs are to

i. Provide growth factors required for maturation of lymphocytes.

ii. Present self antigens for recognition and selection of maturing lymphocytes.

Bone Marrow

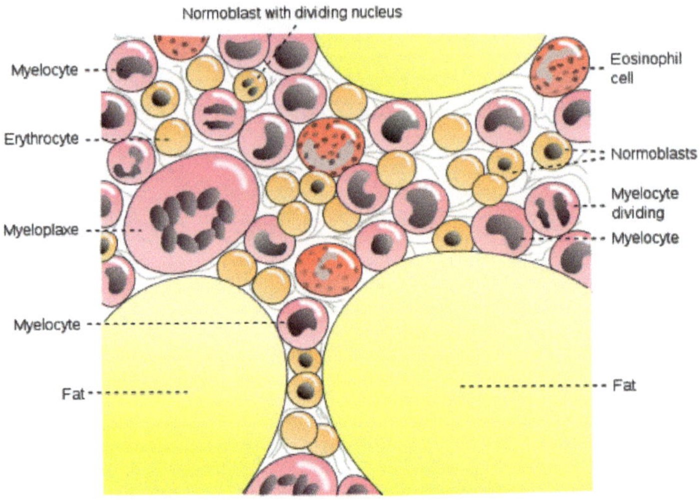

A simplified illustration of cells in bone marrow

Bone marrow is the flexible tissue in the interior of bones. In humans, red blood cells are produced by cores of bone marrow in the heads of long bones in a process known as hematopoiesis. On average, bone marrow constitutes 4% of the total body mass of humans; in an adult having 65 kilograms of mass (143 lbs), bone marrow typically accounts for approximately 2.6 kilograms (5.7 lb). The hematopoietic component of bone marrow produces approximately 500 billion blood cells per day, which use the bone marrow vasculature as a conduit to the body's systemic circulation. Bone marrow is also a key component of the lymphatic system, producing the lymphocytes that support the body's immune system.

Bone marrow transplants can be conducted to treat severe diseases of the bone marrow, including certain forms of cancer such as leukemia. Additionally, bone marrow stem cells have been successfully transformed into functional neural cells, and can also potentially be used to treat illnesses such as inflammatory bowel disease.

Structure

Types of Bone Marrow

The two types of bone marrow are "red marrow", which consists mainly of hematopoietic tissue, and "yellow marrow", which is mainly made up of fat cells. Red blood cells, platelets, and most white blood cells arise in red marrow. Both types of bone marrow contain numerous blood vessels and capillaries. At birth, all bone marrow is red. With age, more and more of it is converted to the yellow type; only around half of adult bone marrow is red. Red marrow is found mainly in the flat bones, such as the pelvis, sternum, cranium, ribs, vertebrae and scapulae, and in the cancellous ("spongy") material at the epiphyseal ends of long bones such as the femur and humerus. Yellow marrow is found in the medullary cavity, the hollow interior of the middle portion of short bones. In cases of severe blood loss, the body can convert yellow marrow back to red marrow to increase blood cell production.

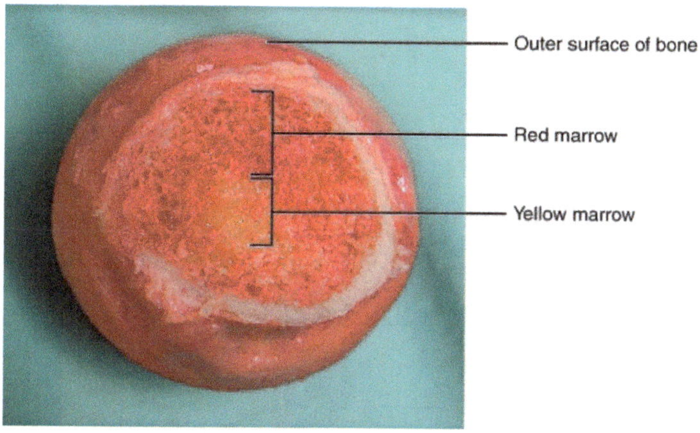

A femoral head with a cortex of bone and medulla of trabecular bone. Both red bone marrow and a central focus of yellow bone marrow are visible.

Stroma

The stroma of the bone marrow is all tissue not directly involved in the marrow's primary function of hematopoiesis. Yellow bone marrow makes up the majority of bone marrow stroma, in addition to smaller concentrations of stromal cells located in the red bone marrow. Though not as active as parenchymal red marrow, stroma is indirectly involved in hematopoiesis, since it provides the hematopoietic microenvironment that facilitates hematopoiesis by the parenchymal cells. For instance, they generate colony stimulating factors, which have a significant effect on hematopoiesis. Cell types that constitute the bone marrow stroma include:

- fibroblasts (reticular connective tissue)
- macrophages, which contribute especially to red blood cell production, as they deliver iron for hemoglobin production.
- adipocytes (fat cells)
- osteoblasts (synthesize bone)
- osteoclasts (resorb bone)
- endothelial cells, which form the sinusoids. These derive from endothelial stem cells, which are also present in the bone marrow.

Cellular Components

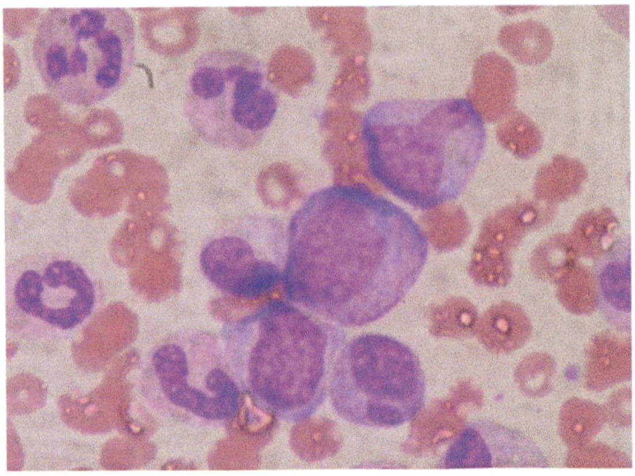

Hematopoietic precursor cells: promyelocyte in the center, two metamyelocytes next to it and band cells from a bone marrow aspirate.

Cellular constitution of the red bone marrow parenchyma			
Group	**Cell type**	**Average fraction**	**Reference range**
Myelopoietic cells	Myeloblasts	0.9%	0.2–1.5
	Promyelocytes	3.3%	2.1–4.1
	Neutrophilic myelocytes	12.7%	8.2–15.7
	Eosinophilic myelocytes	0.8%	0.2–1.3
	Neutrophilic metamyelocytes	15.9%	9.6–24.6
	Eosinophilic metamyelocytes	1.2%	0.4–2.2
	Neutrophilic band cells	12.4%	9.5–15.3
	Eosinophilic band cells	0.9%	0.2–2.4
	Segmented neutrophils	7.4%	6.0–12.0
	Segmented eosinophils	0.5%	0.0–1.3
	Segmented basophils and mast cells	0.1%	0.0–0.2
Erythropoietic cells	Pronormoblasts	0.6%	0.2–1.3
	Basophilic normoblasts	1.4%	0.5–2.4
	Polychromatic normoblasts	21.6%	17.9–29.2
	Orthochromatic normoblast	2.0%	0.4–4.6
Other cell types	Megakaryocytes	< 0.1%	0.0-0.4
	Plasma cells	1.3%	0.4-3.9
	Reticular cells	0.3%	0.0-0.9
	Lymphocytes	16.2%	11.1-23.2
	Monocytes	0.3%	0.0-0.8

In addition, the bone marrow contains hematopoietic stem cells, which give rise to the three classes of blood cells that are found in the circulation: white blood cells (leukocytes), red blood cells (erythrocytes), and platelets (thrombocytes).

Function

Mesenchymal Stem Cells

The bone marrow stroma contains mesenchymal stem cells (MSCs), also known as marrow stromal cells. These are multipotent stem cells that can differentiate into a variety of cell types. MSCs have been shown to differentiate, in vitro or in vivo, into osteoblasts, chondrocytes, myocytes, adipocytes and beta-pancreatic islets cells.

Bone Marrow Barrier

The blood vessels of the bone marrow constitute a barrier, inhibiting immature blood cells from leaving the marrow. Only mature blood cells contain the membrane proteins, such as aquaporin and glycophorin, that are required to attach to and pass the blood vessel endothelium. Hematopoietic stem cells may also cross the bone marrow barrier, and may thus be harvested from blood.

Lymphatic Role

The red bone marrow is a key element of the lymphatic system, being one of the primary lymphoid organs that generate lymphocytes from immature hematopoietic progenitor cells. The bone marrow and thymus constitute the primary lymphoid tissues involved in the production and early selection of lymphocytes. Furthermore, bone marrow performs a valve-like function to prevent the backflow of lymphatic fluid in the lymphatic system.

Compartmentalization

Biological compartmentalization is evident within the bone marrow, in that certain cell types tend to aggregate in specific areas. For instance, erythrocytes, macrophages, and their precursors tend to gather around blood vessels, while granulocytes gather at the borders of the bone marrow.

Society and Culture

Animal bone marrow has been used in cuisine worldwide for millennia, such as the famed Milanese Ossobuco.

Clinical Significance

Disease

The normal bone marrow architecture can be damaged or displaced by aplastic anemia, malignancies such as multiple myeloma, or infections such as tuberculosis, leading to a decrease in the production of blood cells and blood platelets. The bone marrow can also be affected by various forms of leukemia, which attacks its hematologic progenitor cells. Furthermore, exposure to radiation or chemotherapy will kill many of the rapidly dividing cells of the bone marrow, and will therefore result in a depressed immune system. Many of the symptoms of radiation poisoning are due to damage sustained by the bone marrow cells.

To diagnose diseases involving the bone marrow, a bone marrow aspiration is sometimes performed. This typically involves using a hollow needle to acquire a sample of red bone marrow from the crest of the ilium under general or local anesthesia.

Imaging

On CT and plain film, marrow change can be seen indirectly by assessing change to the adjacent ossified bone. Assessment with MRI is usually more sensitive and specific for pathology, particularly for hematologic malignancies like leukemia and lymphoma. These are difficult to distinguish from the red marrow hyperplasia of hematopoiesis, as can occur with tobacco smoking, chronically anemic disease states like sickle cell anemia or beta thalassemia, medications such as granulocyte colony-stimulating factors, or during recovery from chronic nutritional anemias or therapeutic bone marrow suppression. On MRI, the marrow signal is not supposed to be brighter than the adjacent intervertebral disc on T1 weighted images, either in the coronal or sagittal plane, where they can be assessed immediately adjacent to one another. Fatty marrow change, the inverse of red marrow hyperplasia, can occur with normal aging, though it can also be seen with certain treatments such as radiation therapy. Diffuse marrow T1 hypointensity without contrast enhancement or cortical discontinuity suggests red marrow conversion or myelofibrosis. Falsely normal marrow on T1 can be seen with diffuse multiple myeloma or leukemic infiltration when the water to fat ratio is not sufficiently altered, as may be seen with lower grade tumors or earlier in the disease process.

Histology

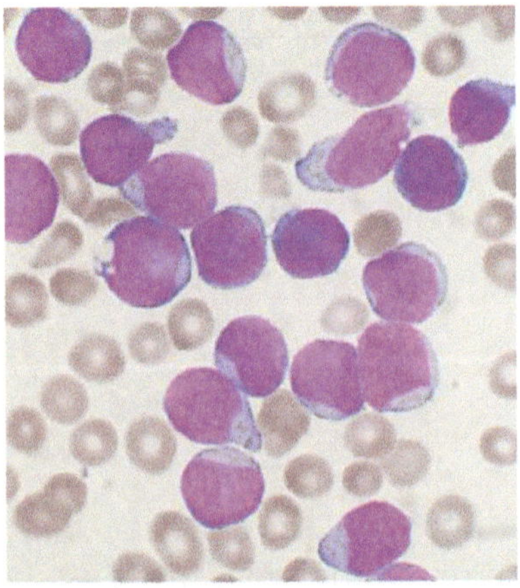

A Wright's-stained bone marrow aspirate smear from a patient with leukemia.

Bone marrow examination is the pathologic analysis of samples of bone marrow obtained via biopsy and bone marrow aspiration. Bone marrow examination is used in the diagnosis of a number of conditions, including leukemia, multiple myeloma, anemia, and pancytopenia. The bone marrow produces the cellular elements of the blood, including platelets, red blood cells and white blood cells. While much information can be gleaned by testing the blood itself (drawn from a vein by phlebotomy), it is sometimes necessary to examine the source of the blood cells in the bone marrow to obtain more information on hematopoiesis; this is the role of bone marrow aspiration and biopsy.

The ratio between myeloid series and erythroid cells is relevant to bone marrow function, and also to diseases of the bone marrow and peripheral blood, such as leukemia and anemia. The normal myeloid-to-erythroid ratio is around 3:1; this ratio may increase in myelogenous leukemias, decrease in polycythemias, and reverse in cases of thalassemia.

Donation and Transplantation

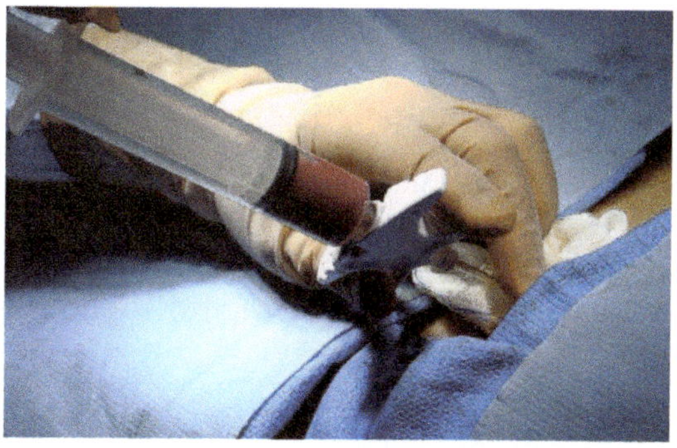

A bone marrow harvest in progress.

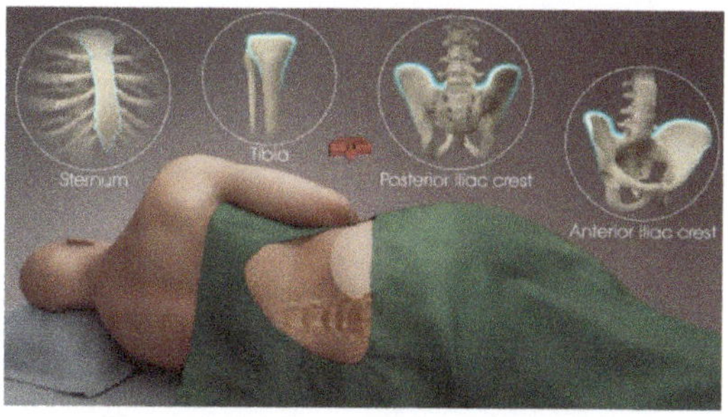

The preferred sites for the procedure

In a bone marrow transplant, hematopoietic stem cells are removed from a person and infused into another person (allogenic) or into the same person at a later time (autologous). If the donor and recipient are compatible, these infused cells will then travel to the bone marrow and initiate blood cell production. Transplantation from one person to another is conducted for the treatment of severe bone marrow diseases, such as congenital defects, autoimmune diseases or malignancies. The patient's own marrow is first killed off with drugs or radiation, and then the new stem cells are introduced. Before radiation therapy or chemotherapy in cases of cancer, some of the patient's hematopoietic stem cells are sometimes harvested and later infused back when the therapy is finished to restore the immune system.

Bone marrow stem cells can be induced to become neural cells to treat neurological illnesses, and can also potentially be used for the treatment of other illnesses, such as inflammatory bowel disease. In 2013, following a clinical trial, scientists proposed that bone marrow transplantation could be used to treat HIV in conjunction with antiretroviral drugs; however, it was later found that HIV remained in the bodies of the test subjects.

Harvesting

The stem cells are typically harvested directly from the red marrow in the iliac crest, often under general anesthesia. The procedure is minimally invasive and does not require stitches afterwards. Depending on the donor's health and reaction to the procedure, the actual harvesting can be an outpatient procedure, or can require 1–2 days of recovery in the hospital.

Another option is to administer certain drugs that stimulate the release of stem cells from the bone marrow into circulating blood. An intravenous catheter is inserted into the donor's arm, and the stem cells are then filtered out of the blood. This procedure is similar to that used in blood or platelet donation. In adults, bone marrow may also be taken from the sternum, while the tibia is often used when taking samples from infants. In newborns, stem cells may be retrieved from the umbilical cord.

Fossil Record

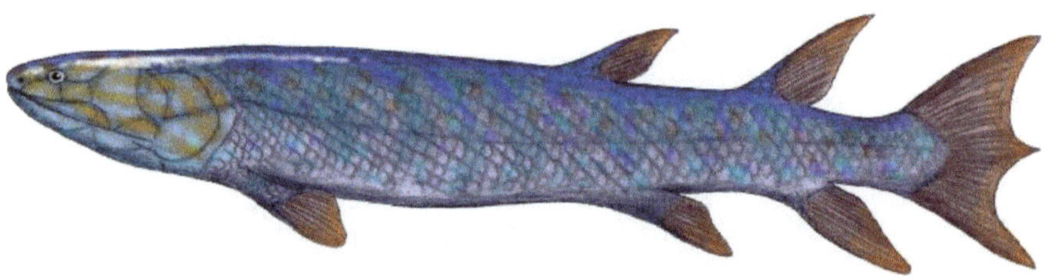

Bone marrow may have first evolved in *Eusthenopteron*, a species of prehistoric fish with close links to early tetrapods.

The earliest fossilised evidence of bone marrow was discovered in 2014 in *Eusthenopteron*, a lobe-finned fish which lived during the Devonian period approximately 370 million years ago. Scientists from Uppsala University and the European Synchrotron Radiation Facility used X-ray synchrotron microtomography to study the fossilised interior of the skeleton's humerus, finding organised tubular structures akin to modern vertebrate bone marrow. *Eusthenopteron* is closely related to the early tetrapods, which ultimately evolved into the land-dwelling mammals and lizards of the present day.

Thymus

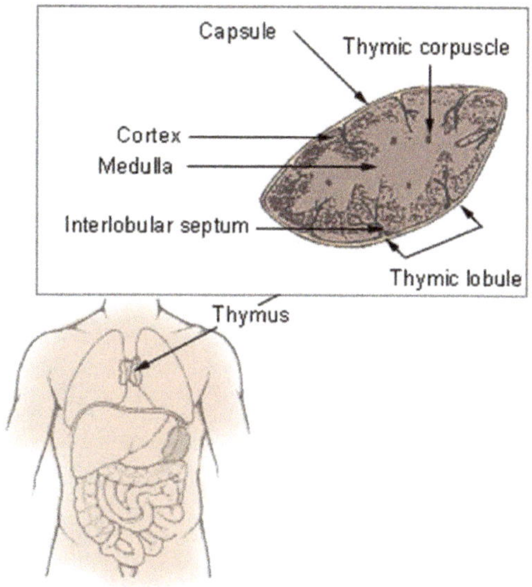

Thymus

The thymus is a specialized primary lymphoid organ of the immune system. Within the thymus, T cells or T lymphocytes mature. T cells are critical to the adaptive immune system, where the body adapts specifically to foreign invaders. The thymus is composed of two identical lobes and is located anatomically in the anterior superior mediastinum, in front of the heart and behind the sternum. Histologically, each lobe of the thymus can be divided into a central medulla and a peripheral cortex which is surrounded by an outer capsule. The cortex and medulla play different roles in the development of T-cells. Cells in the thymus can be divided into thymic stromal cells and cells of hematopoietic origin (derived from bone marrow resident hematopoietic stem cells). Developing T-cells are referred to as thymocytes and are of hematopoietic origin. Stromal cells include epithelial cells of the thymic cortex and medulla, and dendritic cells.

The thymus provides an inductive environment for development of T cells from hematopoietic progenitor cells. In addition, thymic stromal cells allow for the selection of a functional and self-tolerant T cell repertoire. Therefore, one of the most important roles of the thymus is the induction of central tolerance.

The thymus is largest and most active during the neonatal and pre-adolescent periods. By the early teens, the thymus begins to atrophy and thymic stroma is mostly replaced by adipose (fat) tissue. Nevertheless, residual T lymphopoiesis continues throughout adult life.

Structure

The thymus is of a pinkish-gray color, soft, and lobulated on its surfaces. At birth it is about 5 cm in length, 4 cm in breadth, and about 6 mm in thickness. The organ enlarges during childhood, and atrophies at puberty. Unlike the liver, kidney and heart, for instance, the thymus is at its largest in children. The thymus reaches maximum weight (20 to 37 grams) by the time of puberty. The thymus of older people is scarcely distinguishable from surrounding fatty tissue. As one ages the thymus slowly shrinks, eventually degenerating into tiny islands of fatty tissue. By the age of 75 years, the thymus weighs only 6 grams. In children the thymus is grayish-pink in colour and in adults it is yellow.

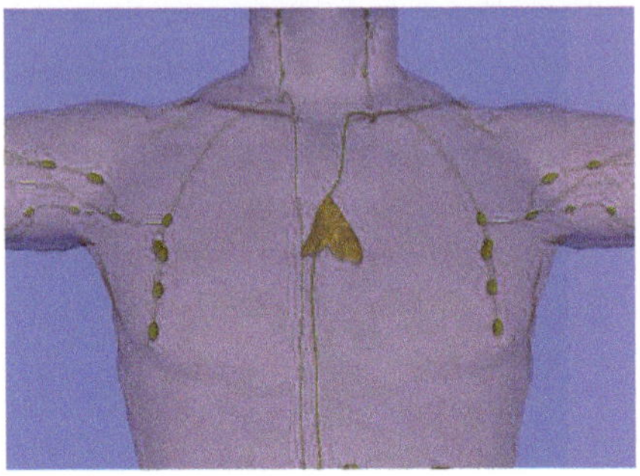

Anterior view of chest showing location and size of adult thymus

If examined when its growth is most active, the thymus will be found to consist of two lateral lobes placed in close contact along the middle line, situated partly in the thorax, partly in the neck, and extending from the fourth costal cartilage upward, as high as the lower border of the thyroid gland. It is covered by the sternum, and by the origins of the sternohyoid and sternothyroid muscles. Below, it rests upon the pericardium, being separated from the aortic arch and great vessels by a layer of fascia. In the neck, it lies on the front and sides of the trachea, behind the sternohyoidei and sternothyreoidei. The two lobes differ slightly in size and may be united or separated.

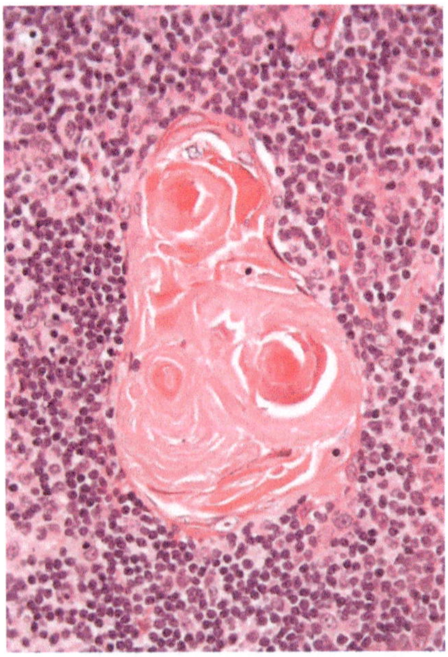

Micrograph showing a thymic corpuscle (Hassall corpuscle), a characteristic histologic feature of the human thymus. H&E stain.

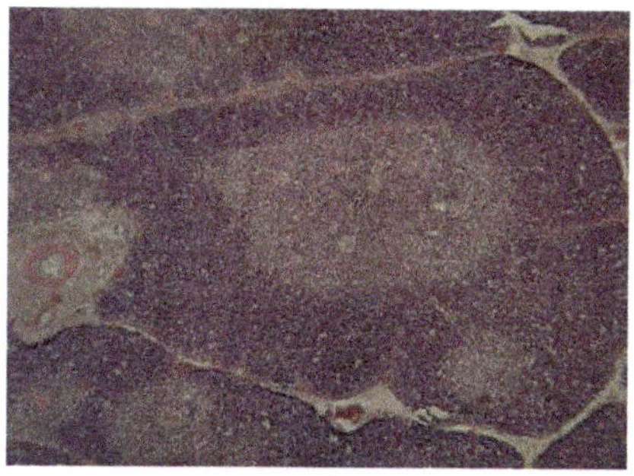

Histology

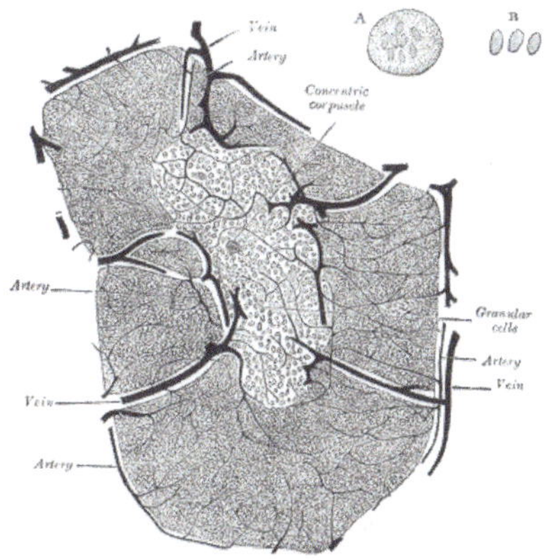

Minute structure of thymus.

Each lateral lobe is composed of numerous lobules held together by delicate areolar tissue; the entire organ being enclosed in an investing capsule of a similar but denser structure. The primary lobules vary in size from that of a pin's head to that of a small pea, and are made up of a number of small nodules or follicles.

The follicles are irregular in shape and are more or less fused together, especially toward the interior of the organ. Each follicle is from 1 to 2 mm in diameter and consists of a medullary and a cortical portion, and these differ in many essential particulars from each other.

Cortex

The cortical portion is mainly composed of lymphocytes, supported by a network of finely-branched epithelial reticular cells, which is continuous with a similar network in the medullary portion. This network forms an adventitia to the blood vessels.

The cortex is the location of the earliest events in thymocyte development, where T cell receptor gene rearrangement and positive selection takes place.

Medulla

In the medullary portion, the network of reticular cells is coarser than in the cortex, the lymphoid cells are relatively fewer in number, and there are concentric, nest-like bodies called Hassall's corpuscles.These concentric corpuscles are composed of a central mass, consisting of one or more granular cells, and of a capsule formed of epithelial cells. They are the remains of the epithelial tubes, which grow out from the third pharyngeal pouches of the embryo to form the thymus. Each follicle is surrounded by a vascular plexus, from which vessels pass into the interior, and radiate from the periphery toward the center, forming a second zone just within the margin of the medullary portion. In the center of the medullary portion there are very few vessels, and they are of minute size.

The medulla is the location of the latter events in thymocyte development. Thymocytes that reach the medulla have already successfully undergone T cell receptor gene rearrangement and positive selection, and have been exposed to a limited degree of negative selection. The medulla is specialized to allow thymocytes to undergo additional rounds of negative selection to remove auto-reactive T-cells from the mature repertoire. Transcriptional regulators AIRE and FEZ2 are expressed by the thymic medullary epithelium, and drives the transcription of organ-specific genes such as insulin to allow maturing thymocytes to be exposed to a more complex set of self-antigens than is present in the cortex.

Blood Supply

The arteries supplying the thymus are derived from the internal thoracic artery, and from the superior thyroid artery and inferior thyroids.

The veins end in the left brachiocephalic vein (innominate vein), and in the thyroid veins.

The nerves are exceedingly minute; they are derived from the vagi and sympathetic nervous system. Branches from the descendens hypoglossi and phrenic reach the investing capsule, but do not penetrate into the substance of the organ.

Development

The two main components of the thymus, the lymphoid thymocytes and the thymic epithelial cells, have distinct developmental origins. The thymic epithelium is the first to develop, and appears in the form of two flask-shape endodermal diverticula, which arise, one on either side, from the third pharyngeal pouch, and extend lateralward and backward into the surrounding mesoderm and neural crest-derived mesenchyme in front of the ventral aorta. Here the thymocytes and epithelium meet and join with connective tissue. The pharyngeal opening of each diverticulum is soon obliterated, but the neck of the flask persists for some time as a cellular cord. By further proliferation of the cells lining the flask, buds of cells are formed, which become surrounded and isolated by the invading mesoderm. Additional portions of thymus tissue are sometimes developed from the fourth pharyngeal pouch.

During the late stages of the development of the thymic epithelium, hematopoietic bone-marrow precursors migrate into the thymus. Normal thymic development thereafter is dependent on the interaction between the thymic epithelium and the hematopoietic thymocytes.

Thymic Involution

The thymus continues to grow between birth and puberty and then begins to atrophy; this thymic involution is directed by the high levels of circulating hormones. Proportional to thymic size, thymic activity (T-cell output) is most active before puberty. Upon atrophy, the size and activity are dramatically reduced, and the organ is primarily replaced with fat (a phenomenon known as "organ involution"). The atrophy is due to the increased circulating level of sex hormones, and chemical or physical castration of an adult results in the thymus increasing in size and activity. Patients with the autoimmune disease myasthenia gravis commonly (70%) are found to have thymic hyperplasia or malignancy. The reason or order of these circumstances has yet to be determined.

Age	Mass
birth	about 15 grams
puberty	about 35 grams
twenty-five years	25 grams
sixty years	less than 15 grams
seventy years	as low as 5 grams

Function

In the two thymic lobes, hematopoietic precursors from the bone-marrow, referred to as thymocytes, mature into T-cells. Once mature, T-cells emigrate from the thymus and constitute the peripheral T-cell repertoire responsible for directing many facets of the adaptive immune system. Loss of the thymus at an early age through genetic mutation (as in DiGeorge Syndrome) results in severe immunodeficiency and subsequent high susceptibility to infection.

Each T cell attacks a specific foreign substance which it identifies with its receptor. T cells have receptors which are generated by randomly shuffling gene segments. Each T cell attacks a different antigen. T cells that attack the body's own proteins are eliminated in the thymus. Thymic epithelial cells express major proteins from elsewhere in the body. First, T cells undergo "Positive Selection", whereby the cell comes in contact with self-MHC, expressed by thymic epithelial cells; those with no interaction are destroyed. Second, the T cell undergoes "Negative Selection" by interacting with thymic dendritic cells, whereby T cells with high affinity interaction are eliminated through apoptosis (to avoid autoimmunity), and those with intermediate affinity survive.

The stock of T-lymphocytes is built up in early life, so the function of the thymus is diminished in adults. It is largely degenerated in elderly adults and is barely identifiable, consisting mostly of fatty tissue. Involution of the thymus has been linked to loss of immune function in the elderly, susceptibility to infection and to cancer.

The ability of T cells to recognize foreign antigens is mediated by the T-cell receptor. The T-cell receptor undergoes genetic rearrangement during thymocyte maturation, resulting in each T-cell bearing a unique T-cell receptor, specific to a limited set of peptide:MHC combinations. The random nature of the genetic rearrangement results in a requirement of central tolerance mechanisms to remove or inactivate those T cells which bear a T-cell receptor with the ability to recognise self-peptides.

1. A rare population of hematopoietic progenitor cells enter the thymus from the blood, and expands by cell division to generate a large population of immature thymocytes.
2. Immature thymocytes each make distinct T-cell receptors by a process of gene rearrangement. This process is error-prone, and some thymocytes fail to make functional T-cell receptors, whereas other thymocytes make T-cell receptors that are autoreactive.
3. Immature thymocytes undergo a process of selection, based on the specificity of their T-cell receptors. This involves selection of T-cells that are *functional (positive selection)*, and elimination of T-cells that are *autoreactive (negative selection)*. The medulla of the thymus is the site of T Cell maturation.

type:	**functional (positive selection)**	**autoreactive (negative selection)**
location:	cortex	medulla
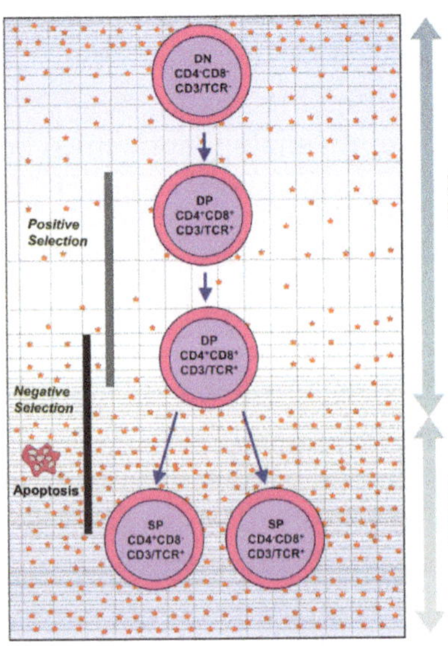	In order to be *positively-selected*, thymocytes will have to interact with several cell surface molecules, MHC/HLA, to ensure reactivity and specificity. Positive selection eliminates (by apoptosis) weakly-binding cells and only takes strongly- or medium-binding cells. (Binding refers to the ability of the T-cell receptors to bind to either MHC class I/II or peptide molecules.)	Negative selection is not 100% complete. Some autoreactive T-cells escape thymic censorship, and are released into the circulation. Additional mechanisms of tolerance active in the periphery exist to silence these cells such as anergy, deletion, and regulatory T cells. If these peripheral tolerance mechanisms also fail, autoimmunity may arise.

Cells that pass both levels of selection are released into the bloodstream to perform vital immune functions.

Clinical Significance

The immune system is a multicomponent interactive system. It effectively protects the host from various infections. An improperly functioning immune system can cause discomfort, disease or even death. The type of malfunction falls into one or more of the following major groups: hypersensitivity or allergy, auto-immune disease, or immunodeficiency.

Hypersensitivity

Allergy results from an inappropriate and excessive immune response to common antigens. Substances that trigger an allergic response are called allergens. Allergies involve mainly IgE, antibodies, and histamine. Mast cells release the histamine. Sometimes an allergen may cause a sudden and severe, possibly fatal reaction in a sensitive individual; this is called anaphylaxis.

Immunodeficiency

As the thymus is the organ of T-cell development, any congenital defect in thymic genesis or a defect in thymocyte development can lead to a profound T cell deficiency in primary immunodeficiency disease. Defects that affect both the T cell and B cell lymphocyte lineages result in Severe Combined Immunodeficiency Syndrome (SCIDs). Acquired T cell deficiencies can also affect thymocyte development in the thymus.

DiGeorge Syndrome

DiGeorge syndrome is a genetic disorder caused by the deletion of a small section of chromosome 22. This results in a midline congenital defect including thymic aplasia, or congenital deficiency of a thymus. Patients may present with a profound immunodeficiency disease, due to the lack of T cells. No other immune cell lineages are affected by the congenital absence of the thymus. DiGeorge syndrome is the most common congenital cause of thymic aplasia in humans. In mice, the nude mouse strain are congenitally thymic deficient. These mice are an important model of primary T cell deficiency.

SCID

Severe combined immunodeficiency syndromes (SCID) are group of rare congenital genetic diseases that result in combined T lymphocyte and B lymphocyte deficiencies. These syndromes are caused by defective hematopoietic progenitor cells which are the precursors of both B- and T-cells. This results in a severe reduction in developing thymocytes in the thymus and consequently thymic atrophy. A number of genetic defects can cause SCID, including IL-7 receptor deficiency, common gamma chain deficiency, and recombination activating gene deficiency. The gene that codes for the enzyme called ADA (adenine deaminase), is located on chromosomes 20.

HIV/AIDS

The HIV virus causes an acquired T-cell immunodeficiency syndrome (AIDS) by specifically killing $CD4^+$ T-cells. Whereas the major effect of the virus is on mature peripheral T-cells, HIV can also infect developing thymocytes in the thymus, most of which express CD4.

Autoimmune Disease

Autoimmune diseases are caused by a hyperactive immune system that instead of attacking foreign pathogens reacts against the host organism (self) causing disease. One of the primary functions of the thymus is to prevent autoimmunity through the process of central tolerance, immunologic tolerance to self antigens.

APECED

Autoimmune polyendocrinopathy-candidiasis-ectodermal dystrophy (APECED) is an extremely rare genetic autoimmune syndrome. However, this disease highlights the importance of the thymus in prevention of autoimmunity. This disease is caused by mutations in the Autoimmune Regulator (AIRE) gene. AIRE allows for the ectopic expression of tissue-specific proteins in the thymus medulla, such as proteins that would normally only be expressed in the eye or pancreas. This expression in the thymus, allows for the deletion of autoreactive thymocytes by exposing them to self-antigens during their development, a mechanism of central tolerance. Patients with APECED develop an autoimmune disease that affects multiple endocrine tissues.

Myasthenia Gravis

Myasthenia gravis is an autoimmune disease caused by antibodies that block acetylcholine receptors. Myasthenia gravis is often associated with thymic hypertrophy. Thymectomy may be necessary to treat the disease.

Cancer

Two primary forms of tumours originate in the thymus.

Thymomas

Tumours originating from the thymic epithelial cells are called thymomas, and are found in about 10-15% of patients with myasthenia gravis. Symptoms are sometimes confused with bronchitis or a strong cough because the tumour presses on the recurrent laryngeal nerve. All thymomas are potentially cancerous, but they can vary a great deal. Some grow very slowly. Others grow rapidly and can spread to surrounding tissues. Treatment of thymomas often requires surgery to remove the entire thymus.

Lymphomas

Tumours originating from the thymocytes are called thymic lymphomas. Lymphomas or leukemias of thymocyte origin are classified as Precursor T acute lymphoblastic leukemia/lymphoma (T-ALL).

People with an enlarged thymus, particularly children, were treated with intense radiation in the years before 1950. There is an elevated incidence of thyroid cancer and leukemia in treated individuals.

Cervical Thymic Cyst

Cervical thymus is a rare malformation. Thymic tissue containing cysts is rarely described in the literature, ectopic glandular tissue included in the wall of cystic formation can trigger a series of problems similar to those of thymus.

Thymic cysts are uncommon lesions, about 150 cases being found. While thymic cyst and ectopic cervical thymus are identified most frequently in childhood, the mean age at which thymoma is diagnosed is 45 years. However, studies have shown the existence necrotic thymic tissue masses in the neck (asymptomatic intravital) more frequently, the incidence reaching nearly 30%. These observations may mean absence of clinical observation.

Thymectomy

Thymectomy is the surgical removal of the thymus. The usual reason for a thymectomy is to gain access to the heart for surgery to correct congenital heart defects in the neonatal period. In neonates, but not older children or adults, the relative size of the thymus obstructs surgical access to the heart. Removal of the thymus in infancy results in immunodeficiency by some measures, although T cells develop compensating function and it remains unknown whether disease incidence in later life is significantly greater. This is because sufficient T cells are generated during fetal life prior to birth. These T cells are long-lived and can proliferate by homeostatic proliferation throughout the lifetime of the patient. However, there is evidence of premature immune aging in patients thymectomized during early childhood.

Other indications for thymectomy include the removal of thymomas and the treatment of myasthenia gravis. Thymectomy is not indicated for the treatment of primary thymic lymphomas. However, a thymic biopsy may be necessary to make the pathologic diagnosis.

Therapeutical Approaches

Thymus Transplantation

A thymus may be transplanted, however, this approach is problematic due to donor requirements and matching tissue with the patient.

Thymus Tissue Engineering

A fully functional thymus derived from reprogrammed mouse embryonic fibroblasts has been grown in the kidney capsule of mice. The newly formed organ resembled a normal thymus histological and molecularly, and upon transplantation it was able to restore immune function in immunocompromised mice. The mouse embryonic fibroblasts were reprogrammed into thymic epithelial cells (TECs) by enforcing the expression of one transcription factor, *FOXN1*.

Society and Culture

When used as food for humans, animal thymic tissue is known as (one of the kinds of) sweetbread.

History

The thymus was known to the ancient Greeks, and its name comes from the Greek word *thumos*, meaning "anger", or "heart, soul, desire, life", possibly because of its location in the chest, near where emotions are subjectively felt; or else the name comes from the herb *thyme*, which became the name for a "warty excrescence", possibly due to its resemblance to a bunch of thyme.

Galen was the first to note that the size of the organ changed over the duration of a person's life.

In the nineteenth century, a fictitious condition known as *status thymicolymphaticus* (an "enlarged" thymus) was erroneously thought to be a cause of Sudden infant death syndrome, causing physicians to recommend radiation therapy as a treatment, a practice that continued into the 1950s.

Due to the large numbers of apoptotic lymphocytes, the thymus was originally dismissed as a "lymphocyte graveyard", without functional importance. The importance of the thymus in the immune system was discovered in 1961 by Jacques Miller, by surgically removing the thymus from one day old mice, and observing the subsequent deficiency in a lymphocyte population, subsequently named T-cells after the organ of their origin. Recently, advances in immunology have allowed the function of the thymus in T-cell maturation to be more fully understood.

Other Animals

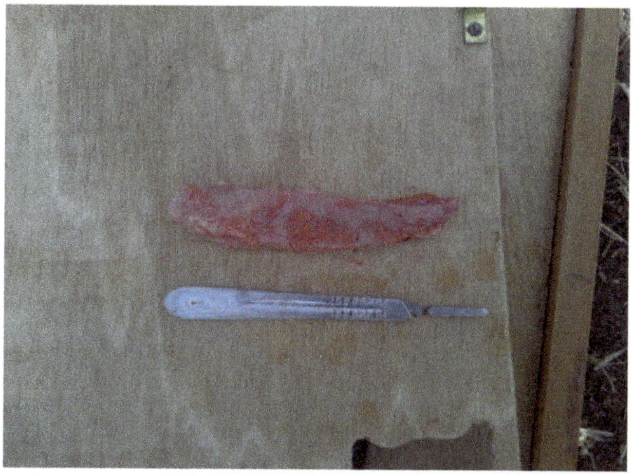

A sheep thymus, several times enlarged, in Peste des petits ruminants

The thymus is present in all jawed vertebrates, where it undergoes the same shrinkage with age and plays the same immunological function as in human beings. Recently, a discrete thymus-like lympho-epithelial structure, termed the thymoid, was discovered in the gills of larval lampreys. Hagfish possess a protothymus associated with the pharyngeal velar muscles, which is responsible for a variety of immune responses. Little is known about the immune mechanisms of tunicates or of *Amphioxus*.

The thymus is also present in most vertebrates, with similar structure and function as the human thymus. Some animals have multiple secondary (smaller) thymi in the neck; this phenomenon has been reported for mice and also occurs in 5 out of 6 human fetuses. As in humans, the Guinea pig's thymus naturally atrophies as the animal reaches adulthood, but the athymic hairless guinea pig (which arose from a spontaneous laboratory mutation) possesses no thymic tissue whatsoever, and the organ cavity is replaced with cystic spaces.

Lymphatic System

The lymphatic system is part of the circulatory system and a vital part of the immune system, comprising a network of lymphatic vessels that carry a clear fluid called lymph (from Latin, *lympha* meaning "water") directionally towards the heart. The lymphatic system was first described in the seventeenth century independently by Olaus Rudbeck and Thomas Bartholin. Unlike the cardiovascular system, the lymphatic system is not a closed system. The human circulatory system processes an average of 20 liters of blood per day through capillary filtration, which removes plasma while leaving the blood cells. Roughly 17 litres of the filtered plasma are reabsorbed directly into the blood vessels, while the remaining three litres remain in the interstitial fluid. One of the main functions of the lymph system is to provide an accessory return route to the blood for the surplus three litres.

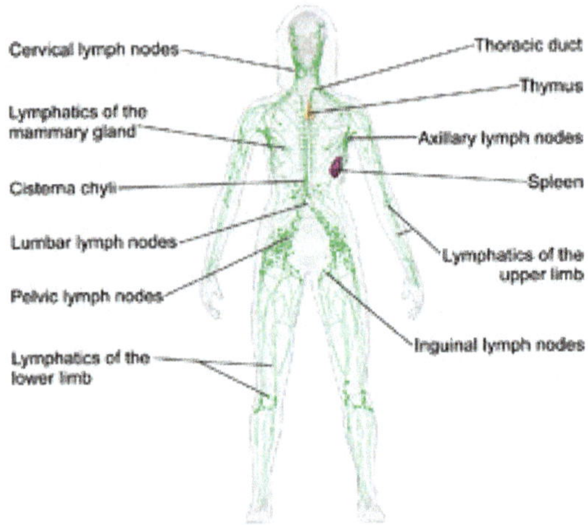

Human lymphatic system

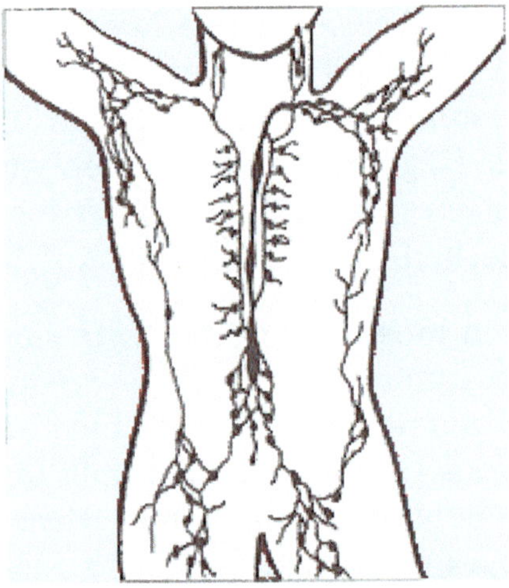

The other main function is that of defense in the immune system. Lymph is very similar to blood plasma: it contains lymphocytes and other white blood cells. It also contains waste products and cellular debris together with bacteria and proteins. Associated organs composed of lymphoid tissue are the sites of lymphocyte production. Lymphocytes are concentrated in the lymph nodes. The spleen and the thymus are also lymphoid organs of the immune system. The tonsils are lymphoid organs that are also associated with the digestive system. Lymphoid tissues contain lymphocytes, and also contain other types of cells for support. The system also includes all the structures dedicated to the circulation and production of lymphocytes (the primary cellular component of lymph), which also includes the bone marrow, and the lymphoid tissue associated with the digestive system.

The blood does not come into direct contact with the parenchymal cells and tissues in the body (except in case of an injury causing rupture of one or more blood vessels), but constituents of the blood first exit the microvascular exchange blood vessels to become interstitial fluid, which comes into contact with the parenchymal cells of the body. Lymph is the fluid that is formed when interstitial fluid enters the initial lymphatic vessels of the lymphatic system. The lymph is then moved along the lymphatic vessel network by either intrinsic contractions of the lymphatic passages or by extrinsic compression of the lymphatic vessels via external tissue forces (e.g., the contractions of skeletal muscles), or by lymph hearts in some animals. The organization of lymph nodes and drainage follows the organization of the body into external and internal regions; therefore, the lymphatic drainage of the head, limbs, and body cavity walls follows an external route, and the lymphatic drainage of the thorax, abdomen, and pelvic cavities follows an internal route. Eventually, the lymph vessels empty into the lymphatic ducts, which drain into one of the two subclavian veins, near their junction with the internal jugular veins.

Structure

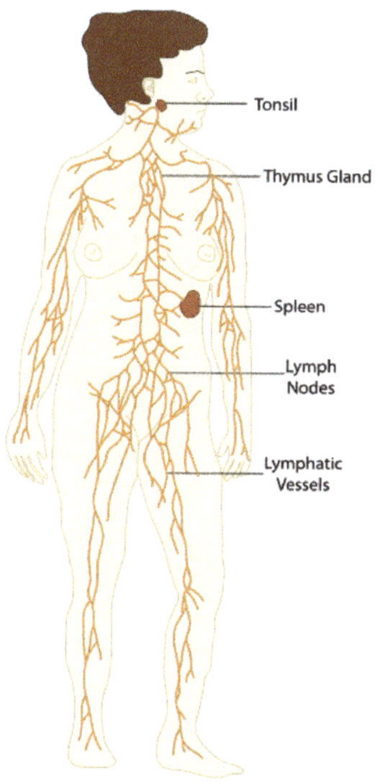

Lymphatic system

The lymphatic system consists of lymphatic organs, a conducting network of lymphatic vessels, and the circulating lymph.

The primary or central lymphoid organs generate lymphocytes from immature progenitor cells.

The thymus and the bone marrow constitute the primary lymphoid organs involved in the production and early clonal selection of lymphocyte tissues. Bone marrow is responsible for both the creation of T cells and the production and maturation of B cells. From the bone marrow, B cells immediately join the circulatory system and travel to secondary lymphoid organs in search of pathogens. T cells, on the other hand, travel from the bone marrow to the thymus, where they develop further. Mature T cells join B cells in search of pathogens. The other 95% of T cells begin a process of apoptosis, a form of programmed cell death.

Secondary or peripheral lymphoid organs, which include lymph nodes and the spleen, maintain mature naive lymphocytes and initiate an adaptive immune response. The peripheral lymphoid organs are the sites of lymphocyte activation by antigens. Activation leads to clonal expansion and affinity maturation. Mature lymphocytes recirculate between the blood and the peripheral lymphoid organs until they encounter their specific antigen.

Secondary lymphoid tissue provides the environment for the foreign or altered native molecules (antigens) to interact with the lymphocytes. It is exemplified by the lymph nodes, and the lymphoid follicles in tonsils, Peyer's patches, spleen, adenoids, skin, etc. that are associated with the mucosa-associated lymphoid tissue (MALT).

In the gastrointestinal wall the appendix has mucosa resembling that of the colon, but here it is heavily infiltrated with lymphocytes.

The tertiary lymphoid tissue typically contains far fewer lymphocytes, and assumes an immune role only when challenged with antigens that result in inflammation. It achieves this by importing the lymphocytes from blood and lymph.)

Lymphoid Tissue

Thymus

The thymus is a primary lymphoid organ and the site of maturation for T cells, the lymphocytes of the adaptive immune system. The thymus increases in size from birth in response to postnatal antigen stimulation, then to puberty and regresses thereafter. The loss or lack of the thymus results in severe immunodeficiency and subsequent high susceptibility to infection. In most species, the thymus consists of lobules divided by septa which are made up of epithelium and is therefore an epithelial organ. T cells mature from thymocytes, proliferate and undergo selection process in the thymic cortex before entering the medulla to interact with epithelial cells.

The thymus provides an inductive environment for development of T cells from hematopoietic progenitor cells. In addition, thymic stromal cells allow for the selection of a functional and self-tolerant T cell repertoire. Therefore, one of the most important roles of the thymus is the induction of central tolerance.

The thymus is largest and most active during the neonatal and pre-adolescent periods.

By the early teens, the thymus begins to atrophy and thymic stroma is mostly replaced by adipose tissue. Nevertheless, residual T lymphopoiesis continues throughout adult life.

Spleen

The main functions of the spleen are:

1. to produce immune response against blood-borne antigens
2. to remove particulate matter and aged blood cells, mainly erythrocytes
3. to produce blood cells during fetal life

The spleen synthesizes antibodies in its white pulp and removes antibody-coated bacteria and antibody-coated blood cells by way of blood and lymph node circulation. A study published in 2009 using mice found that the spleen contains, in its reserve, half of the body's monocytes within the red pulp. These monocytes, upon moving to injured tissue (such as the heart), turn into dendritic cells and macrophages while promoting tissue healing. The spleen is a center of activity of the mononuclear phagocyte system and can be considered analogous to a large lymph node, as its absence causes a predisposition to certain infections.

Like the thymus, the spleen has only efferent lymphatic vessels. Both the short gastric arteries and the splenic artery supply it with blood.

The germinal centers are supplied by arterioles called *penicilliary radicles*.

Up to the fifth month of prenatal development the spleen creates red blood cells. After birth the bone marrow is solely responsible for hematopoiesis. As a major lymphoid organ and a central player in the reticuloendothelial system, the spleen retains the ability to produce lymphocytes. The spleen stores red blood cells and lymphocytes. It can store enough blood cells to help in an emergency. Up to 25% of lymphocytes can be stored at any one time.

Lymph Nodes

A lymph node is an organized collection of lymphoid tissue, through which the lymph passes on its way back to the blood. Lymph nodes are located at intervals along the lymphatic system. Several afferent lymph vessels bring in lymph, which percolates through the substance of the lymph node, and is then drained out by an efferent lymph vessel. There are between five and six hundred lymph nodes in the human body, many of which are grouped in clusters in different regions as in the underarm and abdominal areas. Lymph node clusters are commonly found at the base of limbs (groin, armpits) and in the neck, where lymph is collected from regions of the body likely to sustain pathogen contamination from injuries.

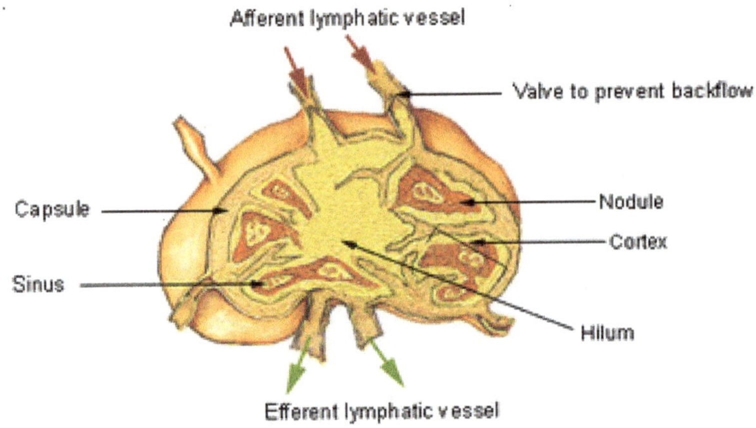

A lymph node showing afferent and efferent lymphatic vessels

The substance of a lymph node consists of lymphoid follicles in an outer portion called the cortex. The inner portion of the node is called the medulla, which is surrounded by the cortex on all sides except for a portion known as the hilum. The hilum presents as a depression on the surface of the lymph node, causing the otherwise spherical lymph node to be bean-shaped or ovoid. The efferent lymph vessel directly emerges from the lymph node at the hilum. The arteries and veins supplying the lymph node with blood enter and exit through the hilum.

The region of the lymph node called the paracortex immediately surrounds the medulla. Unlike the cortex, which has mostly immature T cells, or thymocytes, the paracortex has a mixture of immature and mature T cells. Lymphocytes enter the lymph nodes through specialised high endothelial venules found in the paracortex.

A lymph follicle is a dense collection of lymphocytes, the number, size and configuration of which change in accordance with the functional state of the lymph node. For example, the follicles expand significantly when encountering a foreign antigen. The selection of B cells, or *B lymphocytes*, occurs in the germinal center of the lymph nodes.

Lymph nodes are particularly numerous in the mediastinum in the chest, neck, pelvis, axilla, inguinal region, and in association with the blood vessels of the intestines.

Other Lymphoid Tissue

Lymphoid tissue associated with the lymphatic system is concerned with immune functions in defending the body against infections and the spread of tumors. It consists of connective tissue formed of reticular fibers, with various types of leukocytes, (white blood cells), mostly lymphocytes enmeshed in it, through which the lymph passes. Regions of the lymphoid tissue that are densely packed with lymphocytes are known as *lymphoid follicles*. Lymphoid tissue can either be structurally well organized as lymph nodes or may consist of loosely organized lymphoid follicles known as the mucosa-associated lymphoid tissue.

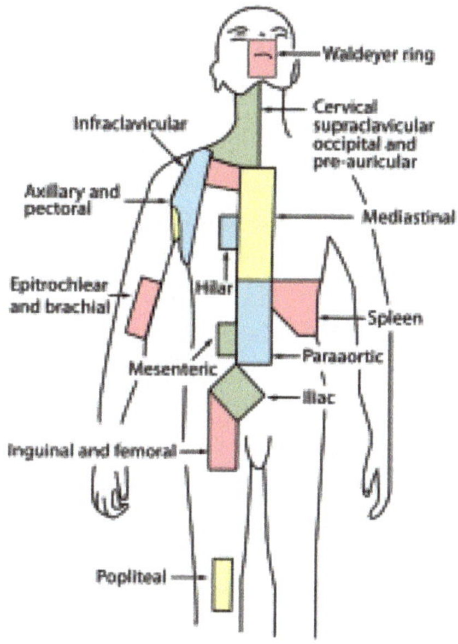

Regional lymph nodes

The central nervous system also has lymphatic vessels, as discovered by University of Virginia Researchers. The search for T-cell gateways into and out of the meninges uncovered functional lymphatic vessels lining the dural sinuses, anatomically integrated into the membrane surrounding the brain.

Lymphatics

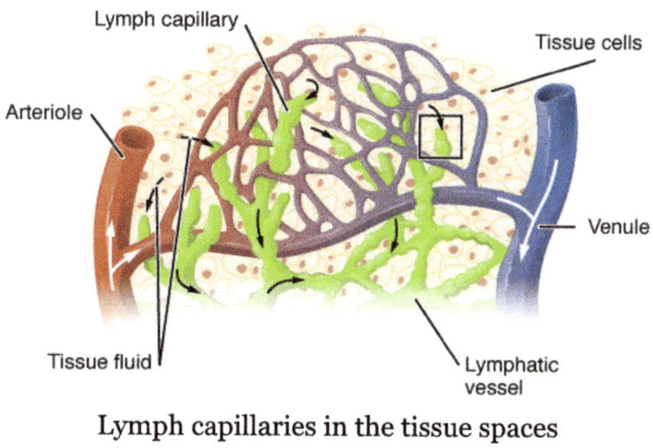

Lymph capillaries in the tissue spaces

The lymphatic vessels, also called lymph vessels, conduct lymph between different parts of the body. They include the tubular vessels of the lymph capillaries, and the larger collecting vessels–the right lymphatic duct and the thoracic duct (the left lymphatic duct). The lymph capillaries are mainly responsible for the absorption of interstitial fluid from the tissues, while lymph vessels propel the absorbed fluid forward into the larger collecting ducts, where it ultimately returns to the bloodstream via one of the subclavian veins. These vessels are also called the lymphatic channels or simply *lymphatics*.

The lymphatics are responsible for maintaining the balance of the body fluids. Its network of capillaries and collecting lymphatic vessels work to efficiently drain and transport extravasated fluid, along with proteins and antigens, back to the circulatory system. Numerous intraluminal valves in the vessels ensure a unidirectional flow of lymph without reflux. Two valve systems are used to achieve this one directional flow—a primary and a secondary valve system. The capillaries are blind-ended, and the valves at the ends of capillaries use specialised junctions together with anchoring filaments to allow a unidirectional flow to the primary vessels. The collecting lymphatics, however, act to propel the lymph by the combined actions of the intraluminal valves and lymphatic muscle cells.

Development

Lymphatic tissues begin to develop by the end of the fifth week of embryonic development. Lymphatic vessels develop from lymph sacs that arise from developing veins, which are derived from mesoderm.

The first lymph sacs to appear are the paired jugular lymph sacs at the junction of the internal jugular and subclavian veins. From the jugular lymph sacs, lymphatic capillary plexuses spread to the thorax, upper limbs, neck and head. Some of the plexuses enlarge and form lymphatic vessels in their respective regions. Each jugular lymph sac retains at least one connection with its jugular vein, the left one developing into the superior portion of the thoracic duct.

The next lymph sac to appear is the unpaired retroperitoneal lymph sac at the root of the mesentery of the intestine. It develops from the primitive vena cava and mesonephric veins. Capillary plexuses and lymphatic vessels spread from the retroperitoneal lymph sac to the abdominal viscera and diaphragm. The sac establishes connections with the cisterna chyli but loses its connections with neighboring veins.

The last of the lymph sacs, the paired posterior lymph sacs, develop from the iliac veins. The posterior lymph sacs produce capillary plexuses and lymphatic vessels of the abdominal wall, pelvic region, and lower limbs. The posterior lymph sacs join the cisterna chyli and lose their connections with adjacent veins.

With the exception of the anterior part of the sac from which the cisterna chyli develops, all lymph sacs become invaded by mesenchymal cells and are converted into groups of lymph nodes.

The spleen develops from mesenchymal cells between layers of the dorsal mesentery of the stomach. The thymus arises as an outgrowth of the third pharyngeal pouch.

Function

The lymphatic system has multiple interrelated functions:

- It is responsible for the removal of interstitial fluid from tissues

- It absorbs and transports fatty acids and fats as chyle from the digestive system
- It transports white blood cells to and from the lymph nodes into the bones
- The lymph transports antigen-presenting cells, such as dendritic cells, to the lymph nodes where an immune response is stimulated.

Function of the Fatty Acid Transport System

Lymph vessels called lacteals are present in the lining of the gastrointestinal tract, predominantly in the small intestine. While most other nutrients absorbed by the small intestine are passed on to the portal venous system to drain via the portal vein into the liver for processing, fats (lipids) are passed on to the lymphatic system to be transported to the blood circulation via the thoracic duct. (There are exceptions, for example medium-chain triglycerides are fatty acid esters of glycerol that passively diffuse from the GI tract to the portal system.) The enriched lymph originating in the lymphatics of the small intestine is called chyle. The nutrients that are released to the circulatory system are processed by the liver, having passed through the systemic circulation.

Immune Function

The lymphatic system plays a major role in body's immune system, as the primary site for cells relating to adaptive immune system including T-cells and B-cells. Cells in the lymphatic system react to antigens presented or found by the cells directly or by other dendritic cells. When an antigen is recognized, an immunological cascade begins involving the activation and recruitment of more and more cells, the production of antibodies and cytokines and the recruitment of other immunological cells such as macrophages.

Clinical Significance

The study of lymphatic drainage of various organs is important in the diagnosis, prognosis, and treatment of cancer. The lymphatic system, because of its closeness to many tissues of the body, is responsible for carrying cancerous cells between the various parts of the body in a process called metastasis. The intervening lymph nodes can trap the cancer cells. If they are not successful in destroying the cancer cells the nodes may become sites of secondary tumors.

Lymphadenopathy

Lymphadenopathy refers to one or more enlarged lymph nodes. Small groups or individually enlarged lymph nodes are generally *reactive* in response to infection or inflammation. This is called *local* lymphadenopathy. When many lymph nodes in different areas of the body are involved, this is called *generalised* lymphadenopathy. Generalised lymphadenopathy may be caused by infections such as infectious mononucleosis, tuberculosis and HIV, connective tissue diseases such as SLE and rheumatoid arthritis, and cancers, including both cancers of tissue within lymph nodes, discussed below, and metastasis of cancerous cells from other parts of the body, that have arrived via the lymphatic system.

Lymphedema

Lymphedema is the swelling caused by the accumulation of lymph, which may occur if the lymphatic system is damaged or has malformations. It usually affects limbs, though the face, neck and abdomen may also be affected. In an extreme state, called elephantiasis, the edema progresses to the extent that the skin becomes thick with an appearance similar to the skin on elephant limbs.

Causes are unknown in most cases, but sometimes there is a previous history of severe infection, usually caused by a parasitic disease, such as lymphatic filariasis.

Lymphangiomatosis is a disease involving multiple cysts or lesions formed from lymphatic vessels.

Lymphedema can also occur after surgical removal of lymph nodes in the armpit (causing the arm to swell due to poor lymphatic drainage) or groin (causing swelling of the leg). Treatment is by massage, *and is not permanent*.

Cancer

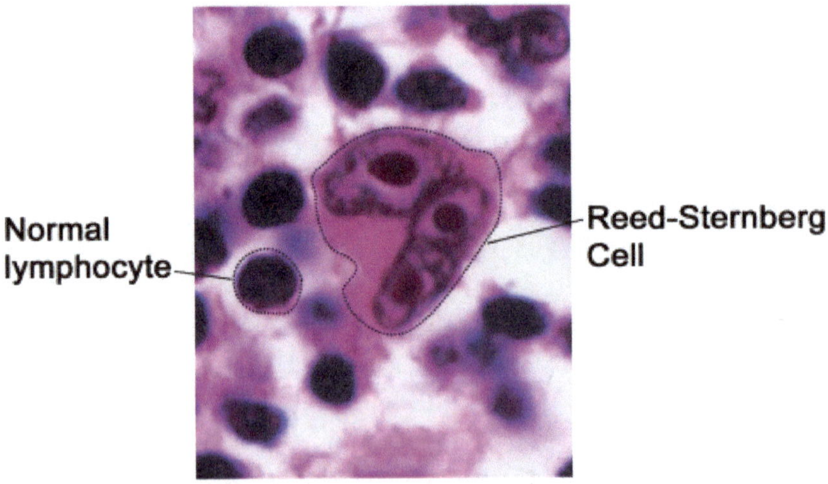

Reed–Sternberg cells.

Cancer of the lymphatic system can be primary or secondary. Lymphoma refers to cancer that arises from lymphatic tissue. Lymphoid leukemias and lymphomas are now considered to be tumors of the same type of cell lineage. They are called “leukemia” when in the blood or marrow and "lymphoma" when in lymphatic tissue. They are grouped together under the name "lymphoid malignancy".

Lymphoma is generally considered as either Hodgkin lymphoma or non-Hodgkin lymphoma. Hodgkin lymphoma is characterised by a particular type of cell, called a Reed–Sternberg cell, visible under microscope. It is associated with past infection with the Epstein-Barr Virus, and generally causes a painless "rubbery" lymphadenopathy. It is staged, using Ann Arbor staging. Chemotherapy generally involves the ABVD and may also involve radiotherapy. Non-Hodgkin lymphoma is a cancer characterised by increased proliferation of B-cells or T-cells, generally occurs in an older age group than Hodgkin lymphoma. It is treated according to whether it is *high-grade* or *low-grade*, and carries a poorer prognosis than Hodgkin lymphoma.

Lymphangiosarcoma is a malignant soft tissue tumor, whereas lymphangioma is a benign tumor occurring frequently in association with Turner syndrome. Lymphangioleiomyomatosis is a benign tumor of the smooth muscles of the lymphatics that occurs in the lungs.

Lymphoid leukemia is another form of cancer where the host is devoid of different lymphatic cells.

Other

- Lymphangitis
- Kikuchi disease
- Chylothorax
- Castleman's disease
- Lymphatic filariasis
- Solitary lymphatic nodule

History

Hippocrates, in 5th century BC, was one of the first people to mention the lymphatic system. In his work *On Joints*, he briefly mentioned the lymph nodes in one sentence. Rufus of Ephesus, a Roman physician, identified the axillary, inguinal and mesenteric lymph nodes as well as the thymus during the 1st to 2nd century AD. The first mention of lymphatic vessels was in 3rd century BC by Herophilos, a Greek anatomist living in Alexandria, who incorrectly concluded that the "absorptive veins of the lymphatics," by which he meant the lacteals (lymph vessels of the intestines), drained into the hepatic portal veins, and thus into the liver. The findings of Ruphus and Herophilos were further propagated by the Greek physician Galen, who described the lacteals and mesenteric lymph nodes which he observed in his dissection of apes and pigs in the 2nd century AD.

In the mid 16th century, Gabriele Falloppio (discoverer of the fallopian tubes), described what are now known as the lacteals as "coursing over the intestines full of yellow matter." In about 1563 Bartolomeo Eustachi, a professor of anatomy, described the thoracic duct in horses as *vena alba thoracis*. The next breakthrough came when in 1622 a physician, Gaspare Aselli, identified lymphatic vessels of the intestines in dogs and termed them *venae alba et lacteae,* which is now known as simply the lacteals. The lacteals were termed the fourth kind of vessels (the other three being the artery, vein and nerve, which was then believed to be a type of vessel), and disproved Galen's assertion that chyle was carried by the veins. But, he still believed that the lacteals carried the chyle to the liver (as taught by Galen). He also identified the thoracic duct but failed to notice its connection with the lacteals. This connection was established by Jean Pecquet in 1651, who found a white fluid mixing with blood in a dog's heart. He suspected that fluid to be chyle as its flow increased when abdominal pressure was applied. He traced this fluid to the thoracic duct, which he then followed to a chyle-filled sac he called the *chyli receptaculum,* which is now known as the cisternae chyli; further investigations led him to find that lacteals' contents enter the venous system via the thoracic duct. Thus, it was proven convincingly that the lacteals did not terminate in the liver, thus disproving Galen's second idea: that the chyle flowed to the liver. Johann Veslingius drew the earliest sketches of the lacteals in humans in 1647.

The idea that blood recirculates through the body rather than being produced anew by the liver and the heart was first accepted as a result of works of William Harvey—a work he published in 1628. In 1652, Olaus Rudbeck (1630–1702), a Swede, discovered certain transparent vessels in the liver that contained clear fluid (and not white), and thus named them *hepatico-aqueous vessels*. He also learned that they emptied into the thoracic duct, and that they had valves. He announced his findings in the court of Queen Christina of Sweden, but did not publish his findings for a year, and in the interim similar findings were published by Thomas Bartholin, who additionally published that such vessels are present everywhere in the body, not just in the liver. He is also the one to have named them "lymphatic vessels." This had resulted in a bitter dispute between one of Bartholin's pupils, Martin Bogdan, and Rudbeck, whom he accused of plagiarism.

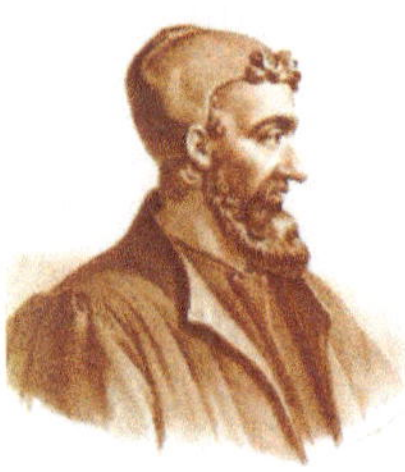

Claude Galien

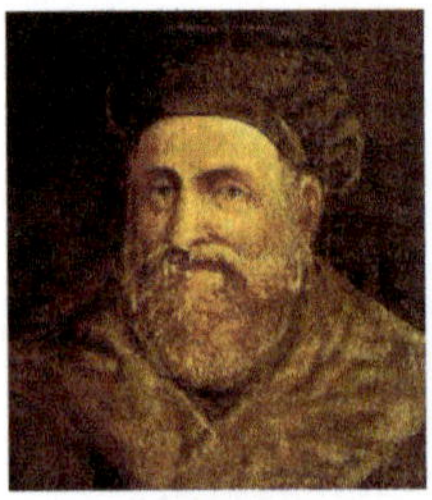

Gabriele Falloppio

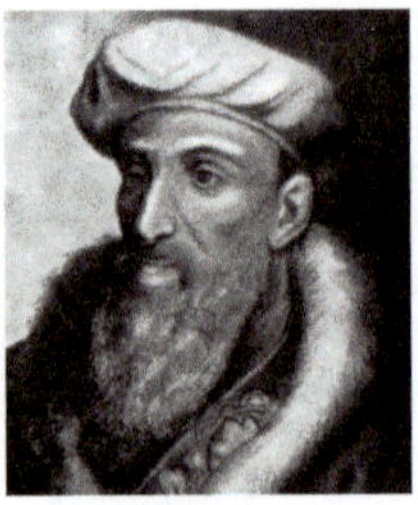

Portrait of Eustachius

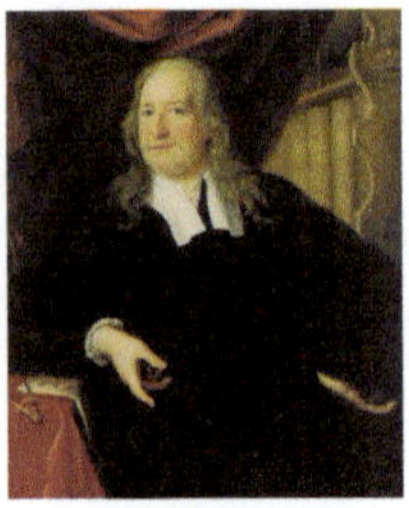

Olaus Rudbeck

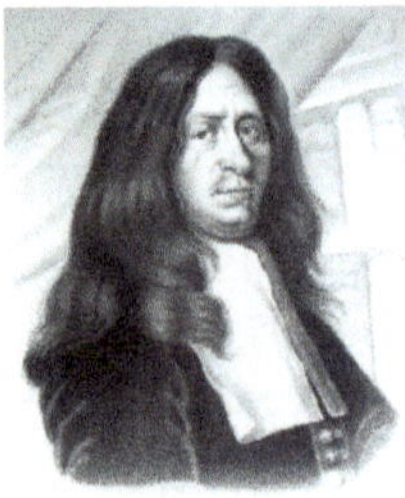

Thomas Bartholin

Galen's ideas prevailed in medicine until the 17th century. It was believed that blood was produced by the liver from chyle contaminated with ailments by the intestine and stomach, to which various spirits were added by other organs, and that this blood was consumed by all the organs of the body. This theory required that the blood be consumed and produced many times over. Even in the 17th century, his ideas were defended by some physicians.

Alexander Monro, of the University of Edinburgh Medical School, was the first to describe the function of the lymphatic system in detail.

Etymology

Lymph originates in the Classical Latin word *lympha* "water", which is also the source of the English word *limpid*.

The adjective used for the lymph-transporting system is *lymphatic*. The adjective used for the tissues where lymphocytes are formed is *lymphoid*. Lymphatic comes from the Latin word *lymphaticus*, meaning "connected to water."

Innate and Adaptive Immunity

Defense against microbes includes an early response action called innate immunity and a later response called as adaptive immunity. Innate immunity is also called natural or native immunity and provides first line of defense against any microbial infection in human body. It usually involves many cellular and biochemical events that react to microbes and their products in order to clear them from the body. The main components of innate immune system are

1) Barriers – skin and outer epithelial surface.
2) Scavenger cells – neutrophils, macrophages, dendritic cell and natural killer cells.
3) Complement system
4) Cytokines
5) Chemical mediators of inflammation

Microbial agents and pathogens contain some molecules over their surface that act as foreign substance for the body and are collectively called as pathogen associated molecular pattern (PAMP). PAMP's are recognized by specific proteins and biochemical molecules produced by cells of innate immunity and these recognition molecules are called as pattern recognition receptors . The innate immune responses are produced against the specific structures present over the microbes and are common to many of them. Thus, they cannot distinguish the minute differences among microbes. In contrast, adaptive immunity is stimulated by constant exposure of infectious agents. The most characteristic feature of adaptive immunity is memory against the repetitive exposure of same pathogen. Furthermore, it has a capacity to distinguish between fine differences among microbes and hence also called as specific immunity . As specific immunity is gathered by constant exposure to the foreign agent, it is better termed as acquired immunity . The central components of adaptive immunity are

1) Lymphocytes and their secreted products e.g. antibodies

2) Foreign substances that trigger specific immune responses and are identified by lymphocytes or antibodies are called as antigens.

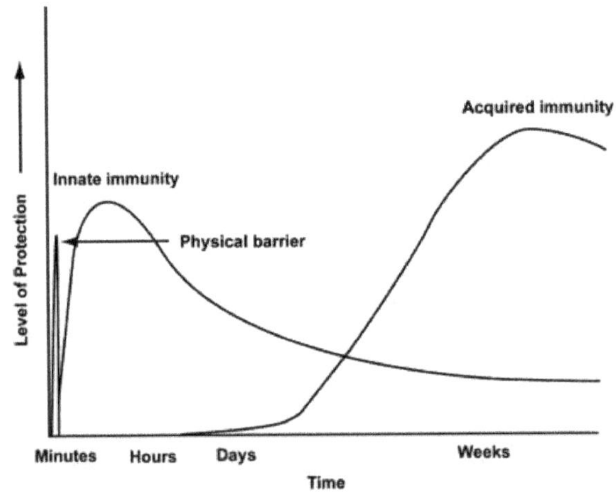

Graph showing the relation between innate and acquired immunity:

Almost all the higher organisms have well developed mechanisms for defending against the microorganisms. Innate and adaptive system work together as they are the components of host integrated system. However there are many microbes that have developed and adapted to resist the innate immunity and hence more robust mechanisms are required for their expulsion. Innate and adaptive immune systems are interlinked; stimulation of anyone against the foreign substances instigates the other and hence functions cooperatively.

Table: common features of innate and adaptive immunity:

Features	Innate	Adaptive
Specificity	Molecules present in a group of related microbes	Microbes and nonmicrobial molecules
Memory	No	Yes
Diversity	Narrow	Wide
Reactivity against self	No	No
Part of innate and adaptive system		
Barrier	Skin, epithelial surface	Lymphocyte and antibodies
Proteins	Complements	Antibodies
Cells	Phagocytes	Lymphocytes

The mechanism of innate immunity provides an initial defense against the infection. Adaptive immune responses develop later and consist of lymphocytes.

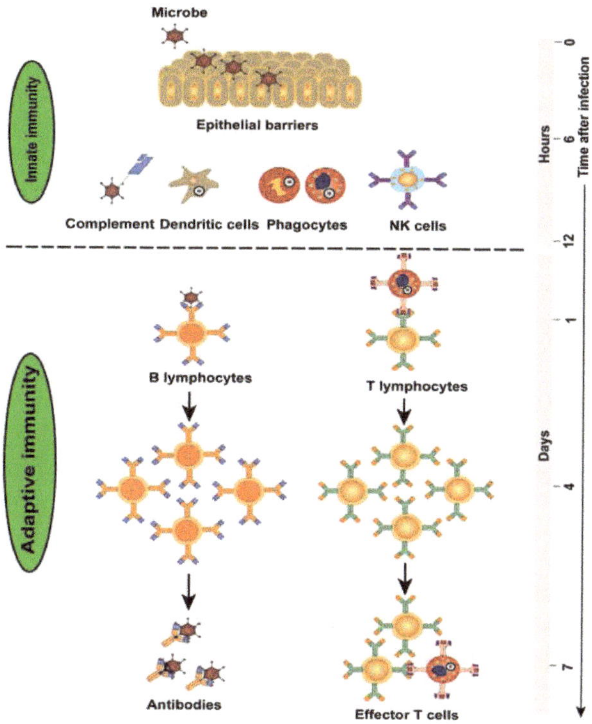

Innate and adaptive immunity:

Complement System

The complement system is a part of the immune system that enhances (complements) the ability of antibodies and phagocytic cells to clear microbes and damaged cells from an organism, promotes inflammation, and attacks the pathogen's plasma membrane. It is part of the innate immune system, which is not adaptable and does not change over the course of an individual's lifetime. It can be recruited and brought into action by the adaptive immune system.

The complement system consists of a number of small proteins found in the blood, in general synthesized by the liver, and normally circulating as inactive precursors (pro-proteins). When stimulated by one of several triggers, proteases in the system cleave specific proteins to release cytokines and initiate an amplifying cascade of further cleavages. The end result of this complement activation or complement fixation cascade is stimulation of phagocytes to clear foreign and damaged material, proxy inflammation to attract additional phagocytes, and activation of the cell-killing membrane attack complex. Over 30 proteins and protein fragments make up the complement system, including serum proteins, serosal proteins, and cell membrane receptors. They account for about 10% of the globulin fraction of blood serum and can serve as opsonins.

Three biochemical pathways activate the complement system: the classical complement pathway, the alternative complement pathway, and the lectin pathway.

History

In 1888, George Nuttall found that sheep blood serum had mild killing activity against the bacterium that causes anthrax. The killing activity disappeared when he heated the blood. In 1891, Hans Ernst August Buchner, noting the same property of blood in his experiments, named the killing property "alexin," which means "to ward off" in Greek. By 1884, several laboratories had demonstrated that serum from guinea pigs that had recovered from cholera killed the cholera bacterium *in vitro*. Heating the serum destroyed its killing activity. Nevertheless, the heat-inactivated serum, when injected into guinea pigs exposed to the cholera bacteria, maintained its ability to protect the animals from illness. Jules Bordet, a young Belgian scientist in Paris at the Pasteur Institute, concluded that this principle has two components, one that maintained a "sensitizing" effect after being heated and one (alexin) whose toxic effect was lost after being heated. The heat-stable component was responsible for immunity against specific microorganisms, whereas the heat-sensitive component was responsible for the non-specific antimicrobial activity conferred by all normal sera. In 1899, Paul Ehrlich renamed the heat-sensitive component "complement."

Ehrlich introduced the term "complement" as part of his larger theory of the immune system. According to this theory, the immune system consists of cells that have specific receptors on their surface to recognize antigens. Upon immunisation with an antigen, more of these receptors are formed, and they are then shed from the cells to circulate in the blood. These receptors, which we now call "antibodies," were called by Ehrlich "amboceptors" to emphasise their bifunctional binding capacity: They recognise and bind to a specific antigen, but they also recognise and bind to the heat-labile antimicrobial component of fresh serum. Ehrlich, therefore, named this heat-labile component "complement," because it is something in the blood that "complements" the cells of the immune system. Ehrlich believed that each antigen-specific amboceptor has its own specific complement, whereas Bordet believed that there is only one type of complement. In the early 20th century, this controversy was resolved when it became understood that complement can act in combination with specific antibodies, or on its own in a non-specific way.

Functions

Complement triggers the following immune functions:

1. Phagocytosis – by opsonizing antigens. C3b has most important opsonizing activity

2. Inflammation – by attracting macrophages and neutrophils
3. Membrane attack – by rupturing cell wall of bacteria

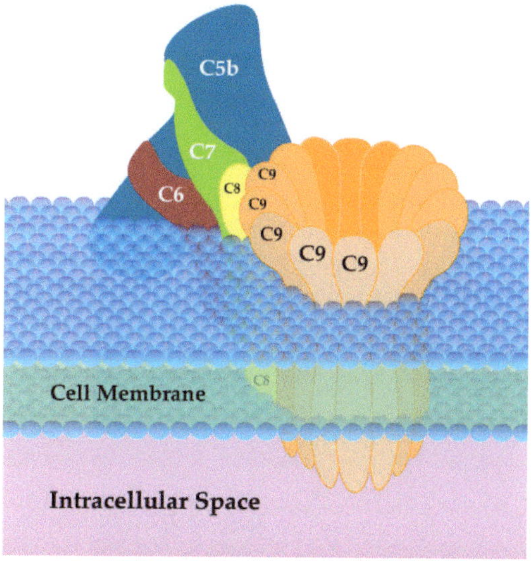

Membrane Attack Complex (Terminal Complement Complex C5b-9)

Overview

Most of the proteins and glycoproteins that constitute the complement system are synthesized by hepatocytes. But significant amounts are also produced by tissue macrophages, blood monocytes, and epithelial cells of the genitourinal tract and gastrointestinal tract. The three pathways of activation all generate homologous variants of the protease C3-convertase. The classical complement pathway typically requires antigen—antibody complexes (immune complexes) for activation (specific immune response), whereas the alternative pathway can be activated by C3 hydrolysis, foreign material, pathogens, or damaged cells. The mannose-binding lectin pathway can be activated by C3 hydrolysis or antigens without the presence of antibodies (non-specific immune response). In all three pathways, C3-convertase cleaves and activates component C3, creating C3a and C3b, and causes a cascade of further cleavage and activation events. C3b binds to the surface of pathogens, leading to greater internalization by phagocytic cells by opsonization.

In the alternative pathway, C3b binds to Factor B. Factor D releases Factor Ba from Factor B bound to C3b. The complex of C3b(2)Bb is a protease which cleaves C5 into C5b and C5a. C5 convertase is also formed by the Classical Pathway when C3b binds C4b and C2a. C5a is an important chemotactic protein, helping recruit inflammatory cells. C3a is the precursor of an important cytokine (adipokine) named ASP (although this is not universally accepted) and is usually rapidly cleaved by carboxypeptidase B. Both C3a and C5a have anaphylatoxin activity, directly triggering degranulation of mast cells as well as increasing vascular permeability and smooth muscle contraction. C5b initiates the membrane attack pathway, which results in the membrane attack complex

(MAC), consisting of C5b, C6, C7, C8, and polymeric C9. MAC is the cytolytic end-product of the complement cascade; it forms a transmembrane channel, which causes osmotic lysis of the target cell. Kupffer cells and other macrophage cell types help clear complement-coated pathogens. As part of the innate immune system, elements of the complement cascade can be found in species earlier than vertebrates; most recently in the protostome horseshoe crab species, putting the origins of the system back further than was previously thought.

Classical Pathway

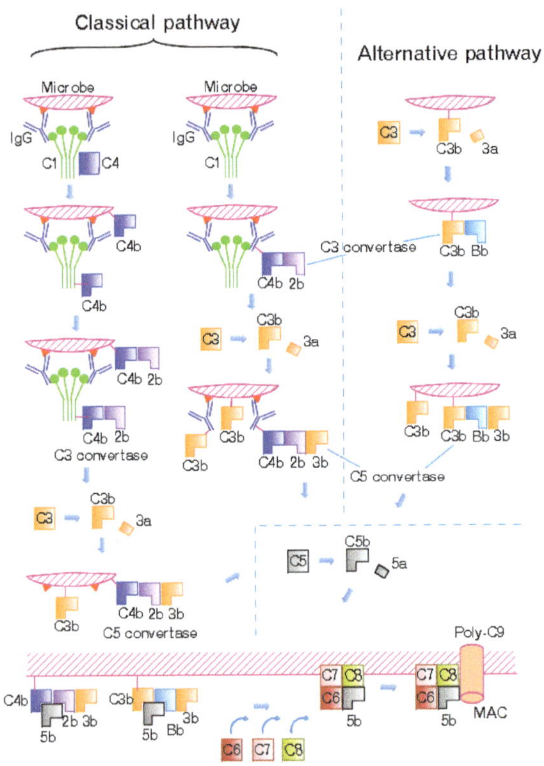

The classical and alternative complement pathways

The classical pathway is triggered by activation of the C1-complex. The C1-complex is composed of 1 molecule of C1q, 2 molecules of C1r and 2 molecules of C1s, or $C1qr^2s^2$. This occurs when C1q binds to IgM or IgG complexed with antigens. A single pentameric IgM can initiate the pathway, while several, ideally six, IgGs are needed. This also occurs when C1q binds directly to the surface of the pathogen. Such binding leads to conformational changes in the C1q molecule, which leads to the activation of two C1r molecules. C1r is a serine protease. They then cleave C1s (another serine protease). The $C1r^2s^2$ component now splits C4 and then C2, producing C4a, C4b, C2a, and C2b. C4b and C2b bind to form the classical pathway C3-convertase (C4b2b complex), which promotes cleavage of C3 into C3a and C3b. C3b later joins with C4b2b to make C5 convertase (C4b2b3b complex).

Alternative Pathway

The alternative pathway is continuously activated at a low level, analogous to a car engine at idle, as a result of spontaneous C3 hydrolysis due to the breakdown of the internal thioester bond (C3 is mildly unstable in aqueous environment). The alternative pathway does not rely on pathogen-binding antibodies like the other pathways. C3b that is generated from C3 by a C3 convertase enzyme complex in the fluid phase is rapidly inactivated by factor H and factor I, as is the C3b-like C3 that is the product of spontaneous cleavage of the internal thioester. In contrast, when the internal thioester of C3 reacts with a hydroxyl or amino group of a molecule on the surface of a cell or pathogen, the C3b that is now covalently bound to the surface is protected from factor H-mediated inactivation. The surface-bound C3b may now bind factor B to form C3bB. This complex in the presence of factor D will be cleaved into Ba and Bb. Bb will remain associated with C3b to form C3bBb, which is the alternative pathway C3 convertase.

The C3bBb complex is stabilized by binding oligomers of factor P (Properdin). The stabilized C3 convertase, C3bBbP, then acts enzymatically to cleave much more C3, some of which becomes covalently attached to the same surface as C3b. This newly bound C3b recruits more B, D and P activity and greatly amplifies the complement activation. When complement is activated on a cell surface, the activation is limited by endogenous complement regulatory proteins, which include CD35, CD46, CD55 and CD59, depending on the cell. Pathogens, in general, don't have complement regulatory proteins (there are many exceptions, which reflect adaptation of microbial pathogens to vertebrate immune defenses). Thus, the alternative complement pathway is able to distinguish self from non-self on the basis of the surface expression of complement regulatory proteins. Host cells don't accumulate cell surface C3b (and the proteolytic fragment of C3b called iC3b) because this is prevented by the complement regulatory proteins, while foreign cells, pathogens and abnormal surfaces may be heavily decorated with C3b and iC3b. Accordingly, the alternative complement pathway is one element of innate immunity.

Once the alternative C3 convertase enzyme is formed on a pathogen or cell surface, it may bind covalently another C3b, to form C3bBbC3bP, the C5 convertase. This enzyme then cleaves C5 to C5a, a potent anaphylatoxin, and C5b. The C5b then recruits and assembles C6, C7, C8 and multiple C9 molecules to assemble the membrane attack complex. This creates a hole or pore in the membrane that can kill or damage the pathogen or cell.

Lectin Pathway

The lectin pathway is homologous to the classical pathway, but with the opsonin, mannose-binding lectin (MBL), and ficolins, instead of C1q. This pathway is activated by binding of MBL to mannose residues on the pathogen surface, which activates the MBL-associated serine proteases, MASP-1, and MASP-2 (very similar to C1r and C1s, respectively), which can then split C4 into C4a and C4b and C2 into C2a and C2b. C4b and C2b then bind together to form the classical C3-convertase, as in the classical pathway. Ficolins are homologous to MBL and function via MASP in a similar way. Several single-nucleotide polymorphisms have been described in M-ficolin in humans, with effect on ligand-binding ability and serum levels. Historically, the larger fragment of C2 was named C2a, but it is now referred to as C2b. In invertebrates without an adaptive immune system, ficolins are expanded and their binding specificities diversified to compensate for the lack of pathogen-specific recognition molecules.

Complement Protein Fragment Nomenclature

Immunology textbooks have used different naming assignments for the smaller and larger fragments of C2 as C2a and C2b. The preferred assignment appears to be that the smaller fragment be designated as C2a: as early as 1994, a well known textbook recommended that the larger fragment of C2 should be designated C2b. However, this was amplified in their 1999 4th edition, to say that: "It is also useful to be aware that the larger active fragment of C2 was originally designated C2a, and is still called that in some texts and research papers. Here, for consistency, we shall call all large fragments of complement b, so the larger fragment of C2 will be designated C2b. In the classical and lectin pathways the C3 convertase enzyme is formed from membrane-bound C4b with C2b."

This nomenclature is used in another literature: The assignment is mixed in the latter literature, though. Some sources designate the larger and smaller fragments as C2a and C2b respectively while other sources apply the converse. However, due to the widely established convention, C2b here is the larger fragment, which, in the classical pathway, forms C4b2b (classically C4b2a). It may be noteworthy that, in a series of editions of Janeway's book, 1st to 7th, in the latest edition they withdraw the stance to indicate the larger fragment of C2 as C2b.

Viral Inhibition

Fixation of the C1a protein on viral surfaces has also been shown to enhance neutralization of viral pathogens.

Review

Activation pathway	Classic	Alternative	Lectin
Activator	Ag-Ab Complex	spontaneous hydrolysis of C3	MBL-Mannose Complex
C3-convertase	C4b2b	C3bBb	C4b2b
C5-convertase	C4b2b3b	C3b3BBb	C4b2b3b
MAC development	C5b+C6+C7+C8+C9		

Activation of Complements by Antigen-associated Antibody

In the classical pathway, C1 binds with its C1q subunits to Fc fragments (made of CH2 region) of IgG or IgM, which has formed a complex with antigens. C4b and C3b are also able to bind to antigen-associated IgG or IgM, to its Fc portion.

Such immunoglobulin-mediated binding of the complement may be interpreted as that the complement uses the ability of the immunoglobulin to detect and bind to non-self antigens as its guiding stick. The complement itself is able to bind non-self pathogens after detecting their pathogen-associated molecular patterns (PAMPs), however, utilizing specificity of antibody, complements are able to detect non-self enemies much more specifically.

Figure shows the classical and the alternative pathways with the late steps of complement activation schematically. Some components have a variety of binding sites. In the classical pathway C4 binds to Ig-associated C1q and $C1r^2s^2$ enzyme cleave C4 to C4b and 4a. C4b binds to C1q, antigen-associated Ig (specifically to its Fc portion), and even to the microbe surface. C3b binds to antigen-associated Ig and to the microbe surface. Ability of C3b to bind to antigen-associated Ig would work effectively against antigen-antibody immune complexes to make them soluble.

Regulation

The complement system has the potential to be extremely damaging to host tissues, meaning its activation must be tightly regulated. The complement system is regulated by complement control proteins, which are present at a higher concentration in the blood plasma than the complement proteins themselves. Some complement control proteins are present on the membranes of self-cells preventing them from being targeted by complement. One example is CD59, also known as protectin, which inhibits C9 polymerisation during the formation of the membrane attack complex. The classical pathway is inhibited by C1-inhibitor, which binds to C1 to prevent its activation.

C3-convertase can be inhibited by Decay accelerating factor (DAF), which is bound to erythrocyte plasma membranes via a GPI anchor.

Role in Disease

Complement Deficiency

It is thought that the complement system might play a role in many diseases with an immune component, such as Barraquer-Simons Syndrome, asthma, lupus erythematosus, glomerulonephritis, various forms of arthritis, autoimmune heart disease, multiple sclerosis, inflammatory bowel disease, paroxysmal nocturnal hemoglobinuria, atypical hemolytic uremic syndrome and ischemia-reperfusion injuries, and rejection of transplanted organs.

The complement system is also becoming increasingly implicated in diseases of the central nervous system such as Alzheimer's disease and other neurodegenerative conditions such as spinal cord injuries.

Deficiencies of the terminal pathway predispose to both autoimmune disease and infections (particularly Neisseria meningitidis, due to the role that the membrane attack complex ("MAC") plays in attacking Gram-negative bacteria).

Infections with *N. meningitidis* and *N. gonorrhoeae* are the only conditions known to be associated with deficiencies in the MAC components of complement. 40-50% of those with MAC deficiencies experience recurrent infections with *N. meningitidis*.

Deficiencies in Complement Regulators

Mutations in the complement regulators factor H and membrane cofactor protein have been associated with atypical hemolytic uremic syndrome. Moreover, a common single nucleotide polymorphism in factor H (Y402H) has been associated with the common eye disease age-related macular degeneration. Polymorphisms of complement component 3, complement factor B, and complement factor I, as well as deletion of complement factor H-related 3 and complement factor H-related 1 also affect a person's risk of developing age-related macular degeneration. Both of these disorders are currently thought to be due to aberrant complement activation on the surface of host cells.

Mutations in the C1 inhibitor gene can cause hereditary angioedema, a genetic condition resulting from reduced regulation of bradykinin by C1-INH.

Paroxysmal nocturnal hemoglobinuria is caused by complement breakdown of RBCs due to an inability to make GPI. Thus the RBCs are not protected by GPI anchored proteins such as DAF.

Diagnostic Tools

Diagnostic tools to measure complement activity include the total complement activity test.

The presence or absence of complement fixation upon a challenge can indicate whether particular antigens or antibodies are present in the blood. This is the principle of the complement fixation test.

Modulation by Infections

Recent research has suggested that the complement system is manipulated during HIV/AIDS to further damage the body.

References

- "HIV Returns in Two Men Thought 'Cured' by Bone Marrow Transplants". RH Reality Check. 10 December 2013. Retrieved 10 December 2013
- Journal of Clinical Investigation. "Evidence of premature immune aging in patients thymectomized during early childhood". JCI. Retrieved 2012-06-11
- Raphael Rubin & David S. Strayer (2007). Rubin's Pathology: Clinicopathologic Foundations of Medicine. Lippincott Williams & Wilkins. p. 90. ISBN 0-7817-9516-8
- "Research Supports Promise of Cell Therapy for Bowel Disease". Wake Forest Baptist Medical Center. 28 February 2013. Retrieved 5 March 2013
- Heppell C1, Richardson G; Roose, T. "A model for fluid drainage by the lymphatic system". Journal. 75 (1): 49–81. doi:10.1007/s11538-012-9793-2. PMID 23161129
- Histology image:07403loa from Vaughan, Deborah (2002). A Learning System in Histology: CD-ROM and Guide. Oxford University Press. ISBN 978-0195151732
- "The Red Cell Membrane: structure and pathologies" (PDF). Australian Centre for Blood Diseases/Monash University. Retrieved 24 January 2015
- Histology image:07401loa from Vaughan, Deborah (2002). A Learning System in Histology: CD-ROM and Guide. Oxford University Press. ISBN 978-0195151732
- National Marrow Donor Program Donor Guide Archived 8 September 2008 at the Wayback Machine. Marrow.org. Retrieved 5 November 2012
- Sapolsky, Robert M. (2004). Why zebras don't get ulcers (3rd ed.). New York: Henry Hold and Co./Owl Books. pp. 182–185. ISBN 0805073698
- MRC, Medical Research Council, (2015-02-12). "Fully functional immune organ grown in mice from lab-created cells". www.mrc.ac.uk. Retrieved 2017-04-07
- Tak W. Mak; Mary E. Saunders (Ph.D.); Mary E. Saunders (2008). Primer to the immune response. Academic Press. pp. 28–. ISBN 978-0-12-374163-9. Retrieved 12 November 2010
- "Spleen: Information, Surgery and Functions". Childrens Hospital of Pittsburgh - Chp.edu. 2010-11-17. Retrieved 2011-04-03
- Blackbourne, Lorne H (2008-04-01). Surgical recall. Lippincott Williams & Wilkins. p. 259. ISBN 978-0-7817-7076-7
- Stanley, Jacqueline (2002-01-01). Essentials of Immunology & Serology. Cengage Learning. p. 103. ISBN 076681064X

2

An Integrated Study of Innate Immune System

The innate immune system is mainly composed of cytokines, complement system, barriers, scavenger cells, and chemical mediators of inflammation. It is the first line of defense against any microbial invasion. They provide a generic defense against pathogens. All the diverse principles of innate immune system have been carefully analyzed in this section.

Innate Immune System

The innate immune system, also known as the non-specific immune system or in-born immunity system, is an important subsystem of the overall immune system that comprises the cells and mechanisms that defend the host from infection by other organisms. The cells of the innate system recognize and respond to pathogens in a generic way, but, unlike the adaptive immune system, the system does not provide long-lasting immunity to the host. Innate immune systems provide immediate defense against infection, and are found in all classes of plant and animal life.

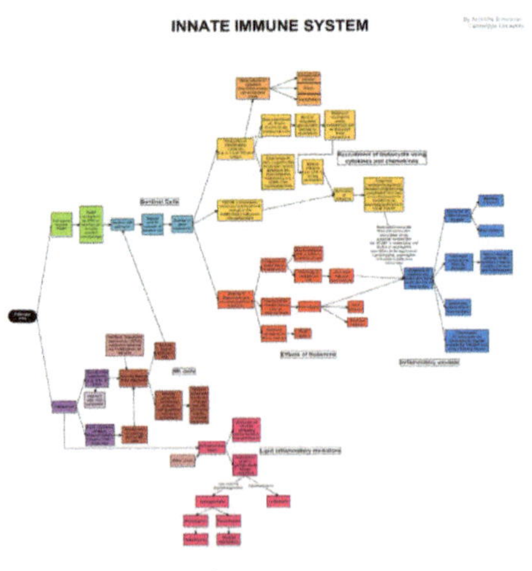

Innate immune system

The innate immune system is an evolutionarily older defense strategy, and is the dominant immune system found in plants, fungi, insects, and primitive multicellular organisms.

The major functions of the vertebrate innate immune system include:

- Recruiting immune cells to sites of infection, through the production of chemical factors, including specialized chemical mediators, called cytokines
- Activation of the complement cascade to identify bacteria, activate cells, and promote clearance of antibody complexes or dead cells
- Identification and removal of foreign substances present in organs, tissues, blood and lymph, by specialized white blood cells
- Activation of the adaptive immune system through a process known as antigen presentation
- Acting as a physical and chemical barrier to infectious agents.

Anatomical Barriers

Anatomical barrier	Additional defense mechanisms
Skin	Sweat, desquamation, flushing, organic acids
Gastrointestinal tract	Peristalsis, gastric acid, bile acids, digestive enzyme, flushing, thiocyanate, defensins, gut flora
Respiratory airways and lungs	Mucociliary elevator, surfactant, defensins
Nasopharynx	Mucus, saliva, lysozyme
Eyes	Tears

Anatomical barriers include physical, chemical and biological barriers. The epithelial surfaces form a physical barrier that is impermeable to most infectious agents, acting as the first line of defense against invading organisms. Desquamation (shedding) of skin epithelium also helps remove bacteria and other infectious agents that have adhered to the epithelial surfaces. Lack of blood vessels and inability of the epidermis to retain moisture, presence of sebaceous glands in the dermis provides an environment unsuitable for the survival of microbes. In the gastrointestinal and respiratory tract, movement due to peristalsis or cilia, respectively, helps remove infectious agents. Also, mucus traps infectious agents. The gut flora can prevent the colonization of pathogenic bacteria by secreting toxic substances or by competing with pathogenic bacteria for nutrients or attachment to cell surfaces. The flushing action of tears and saliva helps prevent infection of the eyes and mouth.

Inflammation

Inflammation is one of the first responses of the immune system to infection or irritation. Inflammation is stimulated by chemical factors released by injured cells and serves to establish a physical barrier against the spread of infection, and to promote healing of any damaged tissue following the clearance of pathogens.

The process of acute inflammation is initiated by cells already present in all tissues, mainly resident macrophages, dendritic cells, histiocytes, Kupffer cells, and mastocytes. These cells present receptors contained on the surface or within the cell, named *pattern recognition receptors* (PRRs), which recognize molecules that are broadly shared by pathogens but distinguishable from host molecules, collectively referred to as pathogen-associated molecular patterns (PAMPs). At the onset of an infection, burn, or other injuries, these cells undergo activation (one of their PRRs recognizes a PAMP) and release inflammatory mediators responsible for the clinical signs of inflammation.

Chemical factors produced during inflammation (histamine, bradykinin, serotonin, leukotrienes, and prostaglandins) sensitize pain receptors, cause local vasodilation of the blood vessels, and attract phagocytes, especially neutrophils. Neutrophils then trigger other parts of the immune system by releasing factors that summon additional leukocytes and lymphocytes. Cytokines produced by macrophages and other cells of the innate immune system mediate the inflammatory response. These cytokines include TNF, HMGB1, and IL-1.

The inflammatory response is characterized by the following symptoms:

- redness of the skin, due to locally increased blood circulation;
- heat, either increased local temperature, such as a warm feeling around a localized infection, or a systemic fever;
- swelling of affected tissues, such as the upper throat during the common cold or joints affected by rheumatoid arthritis;
- increased production of mucus, which can cause symptoms like a runny nose or a productive cough;
- pain, either local pain, such as painful joints or a sore throat, or affecting the whole body, such as body aches; and
- possible dysfunction of the organs or tissues involved.

Immune Response to Microbes

The early innate immune response is the first check point for any microbe that enters the body through different portals (skin, blood, aerosol and mucous membrane). If pathogen enters successfully inside the body the innate immune response counter attacks the pathogens. The major way of innate immunity interventions are inflammation and antiviral defense.

Inflammation

Inflammation is part of the complex biological response of body tissues to harmful stimuli, such as pathogens, damaged cells, or irritants, and is a protective response involving immune cells, blood vessels, and molecular mediators. The function of inflammation is to eliminate the initial cause of cell injury, clear out necrotic cells and tissues damaged from the original insult and the inflammatory process, and to initiate tissue repair.

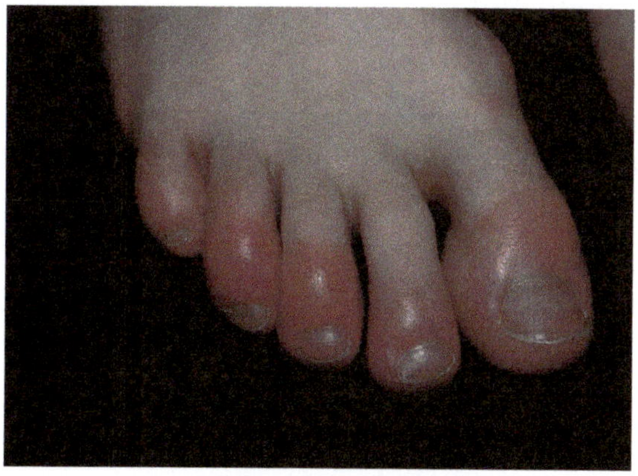

Toes inflamed by chilblains

The classical signs of inflammation are heat, pain, redness, swelling, and loss of function. Inflammation is a generic response, and therefore it is considered as a mechanism of innate immunity, as compared to adaptive immunity, which is specific for each pathogen. Too little inflammation could lead to progressive tissue destruction by the harmful stimulus (e.g. bacteria) and compromise the survival of the organism. In contrast, chronic inflammation may lead to a host of diseases, such as hay fever, periodontitis, atherosclerosis, rheumatoid arthritis, and even cancer (e.g., gallbladder carcinoma). Inflammation is therefore normally closely regulated by the body.

Inflammation can be classified as either *acute* or *chronic*. *Acute inflammation* is the initial response of the body to harmful stimuli and is achieved by the increased movement of plasma and leukocytes (especially granulocytes) from the blood into the injured tissues. A series of biochemical events propagates and matures the inflammatory response, involving the local vascular system, the immune system, and various cells within the injured tissue. Prolonged inflammation, known as *chronic inflammation*, leads to a progressive shift in the type of cells present at the site of inflammation, such as mononuclear cells, and is characterized by simultaneous destruction and healing of the tissue from the inflammatory process.

Inflammation is not a synonym for infection. Infection describes the interaction between the action of microbial invasion and the reaction of the body's inflammatory response — the two components are considered together when discussing an infection, and the word is used to imply a microbial invasive cause for the observed inflammatory reaction. Inflammation on the other hand describes purely the body's immunovascular response, whatever the cause may be. But because of how often the two are correlated, words ending in the suffix *-itis* (which refers to inflammation) are sometimes informally described as referring to infection. For example, the word *urethritis* strictly means only "urethral inflammation", but clinical health care providers usually discuss urethritis as a urethral infection because urethral microbial invasion is the most common cause of urethritis.

It is useful to differentiate inflammation and infection as there are many pathological situations where inflammation is not driven by microbial invasion – for example, atherosclerosis, type III hypersensitivity, trauma, ischaemia. There are also pathological situations where microbial invasion does not result in classic inflammatory response—for example, parasitosis, eosinophilia.

Causes

Physical:

- Burns
- Frostbite
- Physical injury, blunt or penetrating
- Foreign bodies, including splinters, dirt and debris
- Trauma
- Ionizing radiation

Biological:

- Infection by pathogens
- Immune reactions due to hypersensitivity
- Stress

Chemical:

- Chemical irritants
- Toxins
- Alcohol

Psychological:

- Excitement

Types

- Appendicitis
- Bursitis
- Colitis
- Cystitis
- Dermatitis
- Phlebitis
- RSD/CRPS
- Rhinitis
- Tendonitis
- Tonsillitis
- Vasculitis

Comparison between acute and chronic inflammation:

	Acute	**Chronic**
Causative agent	Bacterial pathogens, injured tissues	Persistent acute inflammation due to non-degradable pathogens, viral infection, persistent foreign bodies, or autoimmune reactions
Major cells involved	neutrophils (primarily), basophils (inflammatory response), and eosinophils (response to helminth worms and parasites), mononuclear cells (monocytes, macrophages)	Mononuclear cells (monocytes, macrophages, lymphocytes, plasma cells), fibroblasts
Primary mediators	Vasoactive amines, eicosanoids	IFN-γ and other cytokines, growth factors, reactive oxygen species, hydrolytic enzymes
Onset	Immediate	Delayed
Duration	Few days	Up to many months, or years
Outcomes	Resolution, abscess formation, chronic inflammation	Tissue destruction, fibrosis, necrosis

Cardinal Signs

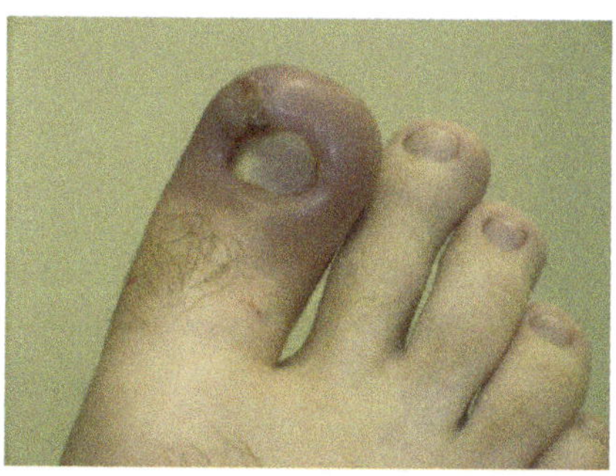

Infected ingrown toenail showing the characteristic redness and swelling associated with acute inflammation

The classic signs and symptoms of acute inflammation:

English	**Latin**
Redness	*Rubor**
Swelling	*Tumor**
Heat	*Calor**
Pain	*Dolor**
Loss of function	*Functio laesa***

All the above signs may be observed in specific instances, but no single sign must, as a matter of course, be present.

These are the original, or "cardinal signs" of inflammation.*

Functio laesa is an apocryphal notion, as it is not unique to inflammation and is a characteristic of many disease states.**

Acute inflammation is a short-term process, usually appearing within a few minutes or hours and begins to cease upon the removal of the injurious stimulus. It involves a coordinated and systemic mobilisation response locally of various immune, endocrine and neurological mediators of acute inflammation. In a normal healthy response, it becomes activated, clears the pathogen and begins a repair process and then ceases. It is characterized by five cardinal signs:

An acronym that may be used to remember the key symptoms is "PRISH", for pain, redness, immobility (loss of function), swelling and heat.

The traditional names for signs of inflammation come from Latin:

- Dolor (pain)
- Calor (heat)
- Rubor (redness)
- Tumor (swelling)
- Functio laesa (loss of function)

The first four (classical signs) were described by Celsus (ca. 30 BC–38 AD), while *loss of function* was added later by Galen even though the attribution is disputed and the origination of the fifth sign has also been ascribed to Thomas Sydenham and Virchow.

Redness and heat are due to increased blood flow at body core temperature to the inflamed site; swelling is caused by accumulation of fluid; pain is due to the release of chemicals such as bradykinin and histamine that stimulate nerve endings. Loss of function has multiple causes.

Acute inflammation of the lung (usually caused in response to pneumonia) does not cause pain unless the inflammation involves the parietal pleura, which does have pain-sensitive nerve endings.

Process of Acute Inflammation

The process of acute inflammation is initiated by resident immune cells already present in the involved tissue, mainly resident macrophages, dendritic cells, histiocytes, Kupffer cells and mast cells. These cells possess surface receptors known as *pattern recognition receptors* (PRRs), which recognize (i.e., bind) two subclasses of molecules: pathogen-associated molecular patterns (PAMPs) and damage-associated molecular patterns (DAMPs). PAMPs are compounds that are associated with various pathogens, but which are distinguishable from host molecules. DAMPs are compounds that are associated with host-related injury and cell damage.

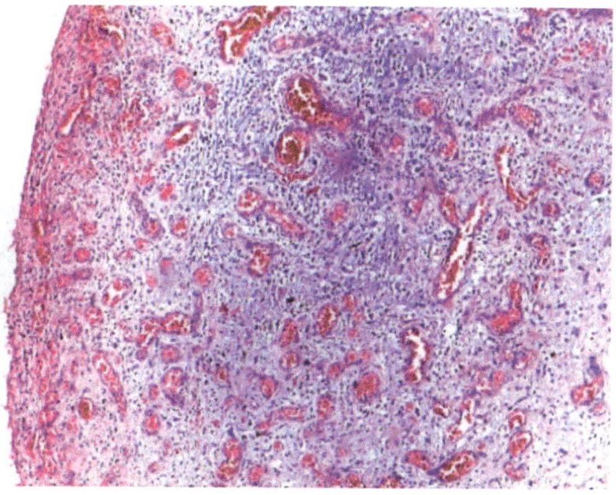

Micrograph showing granulation tissue. H&E stain.

At the onset of an infection, burn, or other injuries, these cells undergo activation (one of the PRRs recognize a PAMP or DAMP) and release inflammatory mediators responsible for the clinical signs of inflammation. Vasodilation and its resulting increased blood flow causes the redness (*rubor*) and increased heat (*calor*). Increased permeability of the blood vessels results in an exudation (leakage) of plasma proteins and fluid into the tissue (edema), which manifests itself as swelling (*tumor*). Some of the released mediators such as bradykinin increase the sensitivity to pain (hyperalgesia, *dolor*). The mediator molecules also alter the blood vessels to permit the migration of leukocytes, mainly neutrophils and macrophages, outside of the blood vessels (extravasation) into the tissue. The neutrophils migrate along a chemotactic gradient created by the local cells to reach the site of injury. The loss of function (*functio laesa*) is probably the result of a neurological reflex in response to pain.

In addition to cell-derived mediators, several acellular biochemical cascade systems consisting of preformed plasma proteins act in parallel to initiate and propagate the inflammatory response. These include the complement system activated by bacteria and the coagulation and fibrinolysis systems activated by necrosis, e.g. a burn or a trauma.

The acute inflammatory response requires constant stimulation to be sustained. Inflammatory mediators are short-lived and are quickly degraded in the tissue. Hence, acute inflammation begins to cease once the stimulus has been removed.

Vascular Component

Vasodilation and Increased Permeability

As defined, acute inflammation is an immunovascular response to an inflammatory stimulus. This means acute inflammation can be broadly divided into a vascular phase that occurs first, followed by a cellular phase involving immune cells (more specifically myeloid granulocytes in the acute setting). The vascular component of acute inflammation involves the movement of plasma fluid, containing important proteins such as fibrin and immunoglobulins (antibodies), into inflamed tissue.

Upon contact with PAMPs, tissue macrophages and mastocytes release vasoactive amines such as histamine and serotonin, as well as eicosanoids such as prostaglandin E2 and leukotriene B4 to remodel the local vasculature. Macrophages and endothelial cells release nitric oxide. These mediators vasodilate and permeabilize the blood vessels, which results in the net distribution of blood plasma from the vessel into the tissue space. The increased collection of fluid into the tissue causes it to swell (edema). This exuded tissue fluid contain various antimicrobial mediators from the plasma such as complement, lysozyme, antibodies, which can immediately deal damage to microbes, and opsonise the microbes in preparation for the cellular phase. If the inflammatory stimulus is a lacerating wound, exuded platelets, coagulants, plasmin and kinins can clot the wounded area and provide haemostasis in the first instance. These clotting mediators also provide a structural staging framework at the inflammatory tissue site in the form of a fibrin lattice – as would construction scaffolding at a construction site – for the purpose of aiding phagocytic debridement and wound repair later on. Some of the exuded tissue fluid is also funnelled by lymphatics to the regional lymph nodes, flushing bacteria along to start the recognition and attack phase of the adaptive immune system.

Acute inflammation is characterized by marked vascular changes, including vasodilation, increased permeability and increased blood flow, which are induced by the actions of various inflammatory mediators. Vasodilation occurs first at the arteriole level, progressing to the capillary level, and brings about a net increase in the amount of blood present, causing the redness and heat of inflammation. Increased permeability of the vessels results in the movement of plasma into the tissues, with resultant *stasis* due to the increase in the concentration of the cells within blood – a condition characterized by enlarged vessels packed with cells. Stasis allows leukocytes to marginate (move) along the endothelium, a process critical to their recruitment into the tissues. Normal flowing blood prevents this, as the shearing force along the periphery of the vessels moves cells in the blood into the middle of the vessel.

Plasma Cascade Systems

- The complement system, when activated, creates a cascade of chemical reactions that promotes opsonization, chemotaxis, and agglutination, and produces the MAC.
- The kinin system generates proteins capable of sustaining vasodilation and other physical inflammatory effects.
- The coagulation system or *clotting cascade*, which forms a protective protein mesh over sites of injury.
- The fibrinolysis system, which acts in opposition to the *coagulation system*, to counterbalance clotting and generate several other inflammatory mediators.

Plasma-derived Mediators

Name	Produced by	Description
Bradykinin	*Kinin system*	A vasoactive protein that is able to induce vasodilation, increase vascular permeability, cause smooth muscle contraction, and induce pain.
C3	*Complement system*	Cleaves to produce *C3a* and *C3b*. C3a stimulates histamine release by mast cells, thereby producing vasodilation. C3b is able to bind to bacterial cell walls and act as an opsonin, which marks the invader as a target for phagocytosis.
C5a	*Complement system*	Stimulates histamine release by mast cells, thereby producing vasodilation. It is also able to act as a chemoattractant to direct cells via chemotaxis to the site of inflammation.
Factor XII (*Hageman Factor*)	*Liver*	A protein that circulates inactively, until activated by collagen, platelets, or exposed basement membranes via conformational change. When activated, it in turn is able to activate three plasma systems involved in inflammation: the kinin system, fibrinolysis system, and coagulation system.
Membrane attack complex	*Complement system*	A complex of the complement proteins C5b, C6, C7, C8, and multiple units of C9. The combination and activation of this range of complement proteins forms the *membrane attack complex*, which is able to insert into bacterial cell walls and causes cell lysis with ensuing bacterial death.
Plasmin	*Fibrinolysis system*	Able to break down fibrin clots, cleave complement protein C3, and activate Factor XII.
Thrombin	*Coagulation system*	Cleaves the soluble plasma protein fibrinogen to produce insoluble fibrin, which aggregates to form a blood clot. Thrombin can also bind to cells via the PAR1 receptor to trigger several other inflammatory responses, such as production of chemokines and nitric oxide.

Cellular Component

The *cellular component* involves leukocytes, which normally reside in blood and must move into the inflamed tissue via *extravasation* to aid in inflammation. Some act as phagocytes, ingesting bacteria, viruses, and cellular debris. Others release enzymatic granules that damage pathogenic invaders. Leukocytes also release inflammatory mediators that develop and maintain the inflammatory response. In general, acute inflammation is mediated by granulocytes, whereas chronic inflammation is mediated by mononuclear cells such as monocytes and lymphocytes.

Leukocyte Extravasation

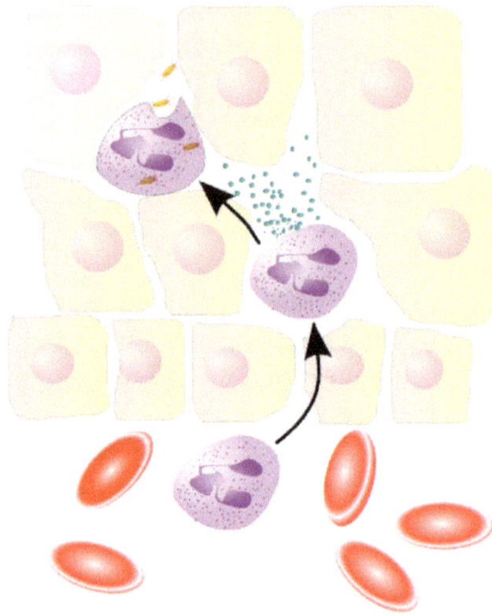

Neutrophils migrate from blood vessels to the infected tissue via chemotaxis, where they remove pathogens through phagocytosis and degranulation

Various leukocytes, particularly neutrophils, are critically involved in the initiation and maintenance of inflammation. These cells must be able to move to the site of injury from their usual location in the blood, therefore mechanisms exist to recruit and direct leukocytes to the appropriate place. The process of leukocyte movement from the blood to the tissues through the blood vessels is known as *extravasation*, and can be broadly divided up into a number of steps:

1. Leukocyte margination and endothelial adhesion: The white blood cells within the vessels which are generally centrally located move peripherally towards the walls of the vessels. Activated macrophages in the tissue release cytokines such as IL-1 and TNFα, which bind to their respective G protein-coupled receptors on the endothelial wall. Signal transduction induces the immediate expression of P-selectin on endothelial cell surfaces. This receptor binds weakly to carbohydrate ligands on the surface of leukocytes and causes them to "roll" along the endothelial surface as bonds are made and broken. Cytokines from injured cells induce the expression of E-selectin on endothelial cells, which functions similarly to P-selectin. Cytokines also induce the expression of integrin ligands such as ICAM-1 and VCAM-1 on endothelial cells, which mediate the adhesion and further slow leukocytes down. These weakly bound leukocytes are free to detach if not activated by chemokines produced in injured tissue. Activation increases the affinity of bound integrin receptors for ICAM-1 and VCAM-1 on the endothelial cell surface, firmly binding the leukocytes to the endothelium.

2. Migration across the endothelium, known as *transmigration*, via the process of diapedesis: Chemokine gradients stimulate the adhered leukocytes to move between adjacent endothelial cells. The endothelial cells retract and the leukocytes

pass through the basement membrane into the surrounding tissue using adhesion molecules such as ICAM-1.

3. Movement of leukocytes within the tissue via chemotaxis: Leukocytes reaching the tissue interstitium bind to extracellular matrix proteins via expressed integrins and CD44 to prevent them from leaving the site. A variety of molecules behave as chemoattractants, for example, C3a or C5, and cause the leukocytes to move along a chemotactic gradient towards the source of inflammation.

Phagocytosis

Extravasated neutrophils in the cellular phase come into contact with microbes at the inflamed tissue. Phagocytes express cell-surface endocytic pattern recognition receptors (PRRs) that have affinity and efficacy against non-specific microbe-associated molecular patterns (PAMPs). Most PAMPs that bind to endocytic PRRs and initiate phagocytosis are cell wall components, including complex carbohydrates such as mannans and β-glucans, lipopolysaccharides (LPS), peptidoglycans, and surface proteins. Endocytic PRRs on phagocytes reflect these molecular patterns, with C-type lectin receptors binding to mannans and β-glucans, and scavenger receptors binding to LPS.

Upon endocytic PRR binding, actin-myosin cytoskeletal rearrangement adjacent to the plasma membrane occurs in a way that endocytoses the plasma membrane containing the PRR-PAMP complex, and the microbe. Phosphatidylinositol and Vps34-Vps15-Beclin1 signalling pathways have been implicated to traffic the endocytosed phagosome to intracellular lysosomes, where fusion of the phagosome and the lysosome produces a phagolysosome. The reactive oxygen species, superoxides and hypochlorite bleach within the phagolysosomes then kill microbes inside the phagocyte.

Phagocytic efficacy can be enhanced by opsonization. Plasma derived complement C3b and antibodies that exude into the inflamed tissue during the vascular phase bind to and coat the microbial antigens. As well as endocytic PRRs, phagocytes also express opsonin receptors Fc receptor and complement receptor 1 (CR1), which bind to antibodies and C3b, respectively. The co-stimulation of endocytic PRR and opsonin receptor increases the efficacy of the phagocytic process, enhancing the lysosomal elimination of the infective agent.

Cell-derived Mediators

Name	Type	Source	Description
Lysosome granules	*Enzymes*	Granulocytes	These cells contain a large variety of enzymes that perform a number of functions. Granules can be classified as either *specific* or *azurophilic* depending upon the contents, and are able to break down a number of substances, some of which may be plasma-derived proteins that allow these enzymes to act as inflammatory mediators.

Histamine	*Monoamine*	Mast cells and basophils	Stored in preformed granules, histamine is released in response to a number of stimuli. It causes arteriole dilation, increased venous permeability, and a wide variety of organ-specific effects.
IFN-γ	*Cytokine*	T-cells, NK cells	Antiviral, immunoregulatory, and anti-tumour properties. This interferon was originally called macrophage-activating factor, and is especially important in the maintenance of chronic inflammation.
IL-8	*Chemokine*	Primarily macrophages	Activation and chemoattraction of neutrophils, with a weak effect on monocytes and eosinophils.
Leukotriene B4	*Eicosanoid*	Leukocytes, cancer cells	Able to mediate leukocyte adhesion and activation, allowing them to bind to the endothelium and migrate across it. In neutrophils, it is also a potent chemoattractant, and is able to induce the formation of reactive oxygen species and the release of lysosomal enzymes by these cells.
LTC4, LTD4	*Eicosanoid*	eosinophils, mast cells, macrophages	These three Cysteine-containing leukotrienes contract lung airways, increase micro-vascular permeability, stimulate mucus secretion, and promote eosinophil-based inflammation in the lung, skin, nose, eye, and other tissues.
5-oxo-eicosatetraenoic acid	*Eicosanoid*	leukocytes, cancer cells	Potent stimulator of neutrophil chemotaxis, lysosome enzyme release, and reactive oxygen species formation; monocyte chemotaxis; and with even greater potency eosinophil chemotaxis, lysosome enzyme release, and reactive oxygen species formation.
5-HETE	*Eicosanoid*	Leukocytes	Metabolic precursor to 5-Oxo-eicosatetraenoic acid, it is a less potent stimulator of neutrophil chemotaxis, lysosome enzyme release, and reactive oxygen species formation; monocyte chemotaxis; and eosinophil chemotaxis, lysosome enzyme release, and reactive oxygen species formation.
Prostaglandins	*Eicosanoid*	Mast cells	A group of lipids that can cause vasodilation, fever, and pain.
Nitric oxide	*Soluble gas*	Macrophages, endothelial cells, some neurons	Potent vasodilator, relaxes smooth muscle, reduces platelet aggregation, aids in leukocyte recruitment, direct antimicrobial activity in high concentrations.
TNF-α and IL-1	*Cytokines*	Primarily macrophages	Both affect a wide variety of cells to induce many similar inflammatory reactions: fever, production of cytokines, endothelial gene regulation, chemotaxis, leukocyte adherence, activation of fibroblasts. Responsible for the systemic effects of inflammation, such as loss of appetite and increased heart rate. TNF-α inhibits osteoblast differentiation.

Morphologic Patterns

Specific patterns of acute and chronic inflammation are seen during particular situations that arise in the body, such as when inflammation occurs on an epithelial surface, or pyogenic bacteria are involved.

- Granulomatous inflammation: Characterised by the formation of granulomas, they are the result of a limited but diverse number of diseases, which include among others tuberculosis, leprosy, sarcoidosis, and syphilis.
- Fibrinous inflammation: Inflammation resulting in a large increase in vascular permeability allows fibrin to pass through the blood vessels. If an appropriate procoagulative stimulus is present, such as cancer cells, a fibrinous exudate is deposited. This is commonly seen in serous cavities, where the conversion of fibrinous exudate into a scar can occur between serous membranes, limiting their function. The deposit sometimes forms a pseudomembrane sheet. During inflammation of the intestine (Pseudomembranous colitis), pseudomembranous tubes can be formed.
- Purulent inflammation: Inflammation resulting in large amount of pus, which consists of neutrophils, dead cells, and fluid. Infection by pyogenic bacteria such as staphylococci is characteristic of this kind of inflammation. Large, localised collections of pus enclosed by surrounding tissues are called abscesses.
- Serous inflammation: Characterised by the copious effusion of non-viscous serous fluid, commonly produced by mesothelial cells of serous membranes, but may be derived from blood plasma. Skin blisters exemplify this pattern of inflammation.
- Ulcerative inflammation: Inflammation occurring near an epithelium can result in the necrotic loss of tissue from the surface, exposing lower layers. The subsequent excavation in the epithelium is known as an ulcer.

Inflammatory Disorders

Inflammatory abnormalities are a large group of disorders that underlie a vast variety of human diseases. The immune system is often involved with inflammatory disorders, demonstrated in both allergic reactions and some myopathies, with many immune system disorders resulting in abnormal inflammation. Non-immune diseases with causal origins in inflammatory processes include cancer, atherosclerosis, and ischaemic heart disease.

A large variety of proteins are involved in inflammation, and any one of them is open to a genetic mutation which impairs or otherwise dysregulates the normal function and expression of that protein.

Examples of disorders associated with inflammation include:

- Acne vulgaris

- Asthma
- Autoimmune diseases
- Autoinflammatory diseases
- Celiac disease
- Chronic prostatitis
- Diverticulitis
- Glomerulonephritis
- Hidradenitis suppurativa
- Hypersensitivities
- Inflammatory bowel diseases
- Interstitial cystitis
- Otitis
- Pelvic inflammatory disease
- Reperfusion injury
- Rheumatic fever
- Rheumatoid arthritis
- Sarcoidosis
- Transplant rejection
- Vasculitis

Atherosclerosis

Atherosclerosis, formerly considered a bland lipid storage disease, actually involves an ongoing inflammatory response. Recent advances in basic science have established a fundamental role for inflammation in mediating all stages of this disease from initiation through progression and, ultimately, the thrombotic complications of atherosclerosis. These new findings provide important links between risk factors and the mechanisms of atherogenesis. Clinical studies have shown that this emerging biology of inflammation in atherosclerosis applies directly to human patients. Elevation in markers of inflammation predicts outcomes of patients with acute coronary syndromes, independently of myocardial damage. In addition, low-grade chronic inflammation, as indicated by levels of the inflammatory marker C-reactive protein, prospectively defines risk of atherosclerotic complications, thus adding to prognostic information provided by traditional risk factors. Moreover, certain treatments that reduce coronary risk also limit inflammation. In the case of lipid lowering with statins, this anti-inflammatory effect does not appear to correlate with reduction in low-density lipoprotein levels. These new insights into inflammation in atherosclerosis not only increase our understanding of this disease but also have practical clinical applications in risk stratification and targeting of therapy for this scourge of growing worldwide importance.

Allergies

An allergic reaction, formally known as type 1 hypersensitivity, is the result of an inappropriate immune response triggering inflammation, vasodilation, and nerve irritation. A common example is hay fever, which is caused by a hypersensitive response by mast cells to allergens. Pre-sensitised mast cells respond by degranulating, releasing vasoactive chemicals such as histamine. These chemicals propagate an excessive inflammatory response characterised by blood vessel dilation, production of pro-inflammatory molecules, cytokine release, and recruitment of leukocytes. Severe inflammatory response may mature into a systemic response known as anaphylaxis.

Other hypersensitivity reactions (*type 2* and *type 3*) are mediated by antibody reactions and induce inflammation by attracting leukocytes that damage surrounding tissue.

Myopathies

Inflammatory myopathies are caused by the immune system inappropriately attacking components of muscle, leading to signs of muscle inflammation. They may occur in conjunction with other immune disorders, such as systemic sclerosis, and include dermatomyositis, polymyositis, and inclusion body myositis.

Leukocyte Defects

Due to the central role of leukocytes in the development and propagation of inflammation, defects in leukocyte functionality often result in a decreased capacity for inflammatory defense with subsequent vulnerability to infection. Dysfunctional leukocytes may be unable to correctly bind to blood vessels due to surface receptor mutations, digest bacteria (Chédiak–Higashi syndrome), or produce microbicides (chronic granulomatous disease). In addition, diseases affecting the bone marrow may result in abnormal or few leukocytes.

Pharmacological

Certain drugs or exogenous chemical compounds are known to affect inflammation. Vitamin A deficiency causes an increase in inflammatory responses, and anti-inflammatory drugs work specifically by inhibiting the enzymes that produce inflammatory eicosanoids. Certain illicit drugs such as cocaine and ecstasy may exert some of their detrimental effects by activating transcription factors intimately involved with inflammation (e.g. NF-κB).

Cancer

Inflammation orchestrates the microenvironment around tumours, contributing to proliferation, survival and migration. Cancer cells use selectins, chemokines and their receptors for invasion, migration and metastasis. On the other hand, many cells of the immune system contribute to cancer immunology, suppressing cancer. Molecular intersection between receptors of steroid hormones, which have important effects on cellular development, and transcription factors that play key roles in inflammation, such as NF-κB, may mediate some of the most critical effects of inflammatory stimuli on cancer cells. This capacity of a mediator of inflammation to influence the effects of steroid hormones in cells, is very likely to affect carcinogenesis on the one hand; on the other hand, due to the modular nature of many steroid hormone receptors, this interaction may offer ways to interfere with cancer progression, through targeting of a specific protein domain in a specific cell type. Such an approach may limit side effects that are unrelated to the tumor of interest, and may help preserve vital homeostatic functions and developmental processes in the organism.

According to a review of 2009, recent data suggests that cancer-related inflammation (CRI) may lead to accumulation of random genetic alterations in cancer cells.

HIV and AIDS

It has long been recognized that infection with HIV is characterized not only by development of profound immunodeficiency but also by sustained inflammation and immune activation. A substantial body of evidence implicates chronic inflammation as a critical driver of immune dysfunction, premature appearance of aging-related diseases, and immune deficiency. Many now regard HIV infection not only as an evolving virus-induced immunodeficiency but also as chronic inflammatory disease. Even after the introduction of effective antiretroviral therapy (ART) and effective suppression of viremia in HIV-infected individuals, chronic inflammation persists. Animal studies also support the relationship between immune activation and progressive cellular immune deficiency: SIVsm infection of its natural nonhuman primate hosts, the sooty mangabey, causes high-level viral replication but limited evidence of disease. This lack of pathogenicity is accompanied by a lack of inflammation, immune activation and cellular proliferation. In sharp contrast, experimental SIVsm infection of rhesus macaque produces immune activation and AIDS-like disease with many parallels to human HIV infection.

Delineating how CD4 T cells are depleted and how chronic inflammation and immune activation are induced lies at the heart of understanding HIV pathogenesis––one of the top priorities for HIV research by the Office of AIDS Research, National Institutes of Health. Recent studies demonstrated that caspase-1-mediated pyroptosis, a highly inflammatory form of programmed cell death, drives CD4 T-cell depletion and inflammation by HIV. These are the two signature events that propel HIV disease progression to AIDS. Pyroptosis appears to create a pathogenic vicious cycle in which dying CD4 T cells and other immune cells (including macrophages and neutrophils) release inflammatory signals that recruit more cells into the infected lymphoid tissues to die. The feed-forward nature of this inflammatory response produces chronic inflammation and tissue injury. Identifying pyroptosis as the predominant mechanism that causes CD4 T-cell depletion and chronic inflammation, provides novel therapeutic opportunities, namely caspase-1 which controls the pyroptotic pathway. In this regard, pyroptosis of CD4 T cells and secretion of pro-inflmammatory cytokines such as IL-1β and IL-18 can be blocked in HIV-infected human lymphoid tissues by addition of the caspase-1 inhibitor VX-765, which has already proven to be safe and well tolerated in phase II human clinical trials. These findings could propel development of an entirely new class of "anti-AIDS" therapies that act by targeting the host rather than the virus. Such agents would almost certainly be used in combination with ART. By promoting "tolerance" of the virus instead of suppressing its replication, VX-765 or related drugs may mimic the evolutionary solutions occurring in multiple monkey hosts (e.g. the sooty mangabey) infected with species-specific lentiviruses that have led to a lack of disease, no decline in CD4 T-cell counts, and no chronic inflammation.

Resolution of Inflammation

The inflammatory response must be actively terminated when no longer needed to prevent unnecessary "bystander" damage to tissues. Failure to do so results in chronic inflammation, and cellular destruction. Resolution of inflammation occurs by different mechanisms in different tissues. Mechanisms that serve to terminate inflammation include:

- Short half-life of inflammatory mediators *in vivo*.
- Production and release of transforming growth factor (TGF) beta from macrophages
- Production and release of interleukin 10 (IL-10)
- Production of anti-inflammatory specialized proresolving mediators, i.e. lipoxins, resolvins, maresins, and neuroprotectins
- Downregulation of pro-inflammatory molecules, such as leukotrienes.
- Upregulation of anti-inflammatory molecules such as the interleukin 1 receptor antagonist or the soluble tumor necrosis factor receptor (TNFR)
- Apoptosis of pro-inflammatory cells
- Desensitization of receptors.

- Increased survival of cells in regions of inflammation due to their interaction with the extracellular matrix (ECM)
- Downregulation of receptor activity by high concentrations of ligands
- Cleavage of chemokines by matrix metalloproteinases (MMPs) might lead to production of anti-inflammatory factors.

> " Acute inflammation normally resolves by mechanisms that have remained somewhat elusive. Emerging evidence now suggests that an active, coordinated program of resolution initiates in the first few hours after an inflammatory response begins. After entering tissues, granulocytes promote the switch of arachidonic acid–derived prostaglandins and leukotrienes to lipoxins, which initiate the termination sequence. Neutrophil recruitment thus ceases and programmed death by apoptosis is engaged. These events coincide with the biosynthesis, from omega-3 polyunsaturated fatty acids, of resolvins and protectins, which critically shorten the period of neutrophil infiltration by initiating apoptosis. As a consequence, apoptotic neutrophils undergo phagocytosis by macrophages, leading to neutrophil clearance and release of anti-inflammatory and reparative cytokines such as transforming growth factor-β1. The anti-inflammatory program ends with the departure of macrophages through the lymphatics. "
>
> —CHARLES SERHAN

Connection to Depression

There is evidence for a link between inflammation and depression. Inflammatory processes can be triggered by negative cognitions or their consequences, such as stress, violence, or deprivation. Thus, negative cognitions can cause inflammation that can, in turn, lead to depression. In addition there is increasing evidence that inflammation can cause depression because of the increase of cytokines, setting the brain into a "sickness mode". Classical symptoms of being physically sick like lethargy show a large overlap in behaviors that characterize depression. Levels of cytokines tend to increase sharply during depressive episodes in manics and drop off during remission. Furthermore, it has been shown in clinical trials that anti-inflammatory medicines taken in addition to antidepressants not only significantly improves symptoms but also increases the proportion of subjects positively responding to treatment. Inflammations that lead to serious depression could be caused by common infections such as those caused by a virus, bacteria or even parasites.

Systemic Effects

An infectious organism can escape the confines of the immediate tissue via the circulatory system or lymphatic system, where it may spread to other parts of the body. If an organism is not contained by the actions of acute inflammation it may gain access to the lymphatic system via nearby lymph vessels. An infection of the lymph vessels is known as lymphangitis, and infection of a lymph node is known as lymphadenitis.

When lymph nodes cannot destroy all pathogens, the infection spreads further. A pathogen can gain access to the bloodstream through lymphatic drainage into the circulatory system.

When inflammation overwhelms the host, systemic inflammatory response syndrome is diagnosed. When it is due to infection, the term sepsis is applied, with the terms bacteremia being applied specifically for bacterial sepsis and viremia specifically to viral sepsis. Vasodilation and organ dysfunction are serious problems associated with widespread infection that may lead to septic shock and death.

Acute-phase Proteins

Inflammation also induces high systemic levels of acute-phase proteins. In acute inflammation, these proteins prove beneficial; however, in chronic inflammation they can contribute to amyloidosis. These proteins include C-reactive protein, serum amyloid A, and serum amyloid P, which cause a range of systemic effects including:

- Fever
- Increased blood pressure
- Decreased sweating
- Malaise
- Loss of appetite
- Somnolence

Leukocyte Numbers

Inflammation often affects the numbers of leukocytes present in the body:

- Leukocytosis is often seen during inflammation induced by infection, where it results in a large increase in the amount of leukocytes in the blood, especially immature cells. Leukocyte numbers usually increase to between 15 000 and 20 000 cells per microliter, but extreme cases can see it approach 100 000 cells per microliter. Bacterial infection usually results in an increase of neutrophils, creating neutrophilia, whereas diseases such as asthma, hay fever, and parasite infestation result in an increase in eosinophils, creating eosinophilia.
- Leukopenia can be induced by certain infections and diseases, including viral infection, *Rickettsia* infection, some protozoa, tuberculosis, and some cancers.

Systemic Inflammation and Obesity

With the discovery of interleukins (IL), the concept of systemic inflammation developed. Although the processes involved are identical to tissue inflammation, systemic inflammation is not confined to a particular tissue but involves the endothelium and other organ systems.

Chronic inflammation is widely observed in obesity. The obese commonly have many elevated markers of inflammation, including:

- IL-6 (Interleukin-6)
- IL-8 (Interleukin-8)
- IL-18 (Interleukin-18)
- TNF-α (Tumor necrosis factor-alpha)
- CRP (C-reactive protein)
- Insulin
- Blood glucose
- Leptin

Low-grade chronic inflammation is characterized by a two- to threefold increase in the systemic concentrations of cytokines such as TNF-α, IL-6, and CRP. Waist circumference correlates significantly with systemic inflammatory response. A predominant factor in this correlation is due to the autoimmune response triggered by adiposity, whereby immune cells may mistake fatty deposits for intruders. The body attacks fat similar to bacteria and fungi. When expanded fat cells leak or break open, macrophages mobilize to clean up and embed into the adipose tissue. Then macrophages release inflammatory chemicals, including TNF-α and (IL-6). TNF's primary role is to regulate the immune cells and induce inflammation. White blood cells then assist by releasing more cytokines. This link between adiposity and inflammation has been shown to produce 10–35% of IL-6 in a resting individual, and this production increases with increasing adiposity.

Loss of white adipose tissue reduces levels of inflammation markers. The association of systemic inflammation with insulin resistance and atherosclerosis is the subject of intense research.

In the obese mouse models, inflammation and macrophage-specific genes are upregulated in white adipose tissue (WAT). There were also signs of dramatic increase in circulating insulin level, adipocyte lipolysis and formation of multinucleate giant cells. The fat-derived protein called angiopoietin-like protein 2 (Angptl2) elevates in fat tissues. Higher than normal Angptl2 level in fat tissues develop inflammation as well as insulin and leptin resistance. Stored fat secretes Leptin to signal satiety. Leptin resistance plays a role in the process where appetite overrules the message of satiety. Angptl2 then starts an inflammatory cascade causing blood vessels to remodel and attract macrophages. Angptl2 is an adipocyte-derived inflammatory mediator linking obesity to systemic insulin resistance. It is possible that, as an inflammatory marker, leptin responds specifically to adipose-derived inflammatory cytokines.

C-reactive protein (CRP) is generated at a higher level in obese people. It raises when there is inflammation throughout the body. Mild elevation in CRP increase risk of heart attacks, strokes, high blood pressure, muscle weakness and fragility.

Systemic Inflammation and Overeating

Hyperglycemia induces IL-6 production from endothelial cells and macrophages. Meals high in saturated fat, as well as meals high in calories have been associated with increases in inflammatory markers. While the inflammatory responses are acute and arise in response to overeating, the response may become chronic if the overeating is chronic.

Bente Klarlund Pedersen wrote in 2013 that interstitial abdominal adiposity (also referred to as accumulated intra-abdominal fat) is a major and possibly primary factor in increasing systemic risk for multiple inflammatory diseases. However, she indicates that this is mediated via TNF-α, rather than Interleukin 6, which she identified as a myokine in 2003. Dr. Pedersen concludes: "Until the beginning of this millennium, it was commonly thought that the increase in IL-6 during exercise was a consequence of an immune response due to local damage in the working muscles and it was hypothesized that macrophages were responsible for this increase. However, an early study demonstrated that IL-6 mRNA in monocytes did not increase as a result of exercise."

Dr. Pedersen continues (in the same article): "Patients with diabetes have a high protein expression of TNF-α in skeletal muscle and increased TNF-α levels in plasma, and it is likely that adipose tissue, which produces TNF-α, is the main source of the circulating TNF-α. In vitro studies demonstrate that TNF-α has direct inhibitory effects on insulin signaling. In addition, TNF-α infusion in healthy humans induces insulin resistance in skeletal muscle, without an effect on EGP [endogenous glucose production]. It has also been proposed that TNF-α causes insulin resistance indirectly *in vivo* by increasing the release of FFAs from adipose tissue. TNF-α increases lipolysis in human and 3T3-L1 adipocytes. However, TNF-α has no effect on muscle fatty acid oxidation, but increases fatty acid incorporation into diacylglycerol, which may be involved in the development of the TNF-α-induced insulin resistance in skeletal muscle. In addition, evidence suggests that TNF-α plays a direct role in linking insulin resistance to vascular disease. Moreover, in CVDs, activated immune cells also play major roles, particularly in the etiology of atherosclerosis. Importantly, also tumor initiation, promotion, and progression is stimulated by systemic elevation of proinflammatory cytokines."

Outcomes

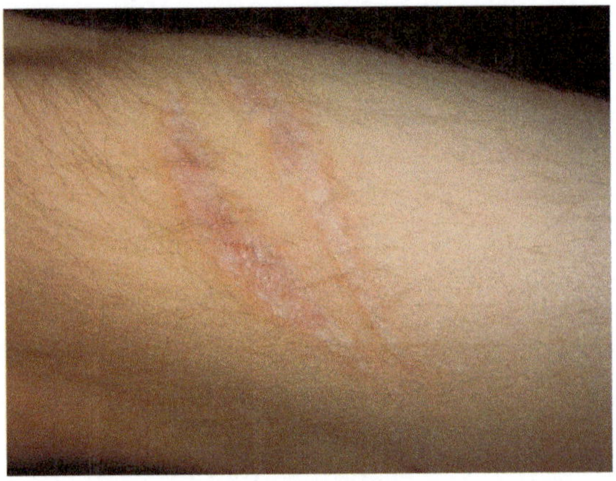

Scars present on the skin, evidence of fibrosis and healing of a wound

The outcome in a particular circumstance will be determined by the tissue in which the injury has occurred and the injurious agent that is causing it. Here are the possible outcomes to inflammation:

1. Resolution

   The complete restoration of the inflamed tissue back to a normal status. Inflammatory measures such as vasodilation, chemical production, and leukocyte infiltration cease, and damaged parenchymal cells regenerate. In situations where limited or short-lived inflammation has occurred this is usually the outcome.

2. Fibrosis

   Large amounts of tissue destruction, or damage in tissues unable to regenerate, cannot be regenerated completely by the body. Fibrous scarring occurs in these areas of damage, forming a scar composed primarily of collagen. The scar will not contain any specialized structures, such as parenchymal cells, hence functional impairment may occur.

3. Abscess formation

   A cavity is formed containing pus, an opaque liquid containing dead white blood cells and bacteria with general debris from destroyed cells.

4. Chronic inflammation

   In acute inflammation, if the injurious agent persists then chronic inflammation will ensue. This process, marked by inflammation lasting many days, months or even years, may lead to the formation of a chronic wound. Chronic inflammation is characterised by the dominating presence of macrophages in the injured tissue. These cells are powerful defensive agents of the body, but the toxins they release (including reactive oxygen species) are injurious to the organism's own tissues as well as invading agents. As a consequence, chronic inflammation is almost always accompanied by tissue destruction.

Examples

Inflammation is usually indicated by adding the suffix "itis", as shown below. However, some conditions such as asthma and pneumonia do not follow this convention.

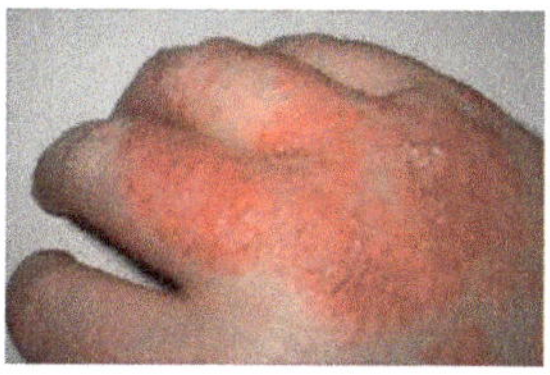

Acute dermatitis

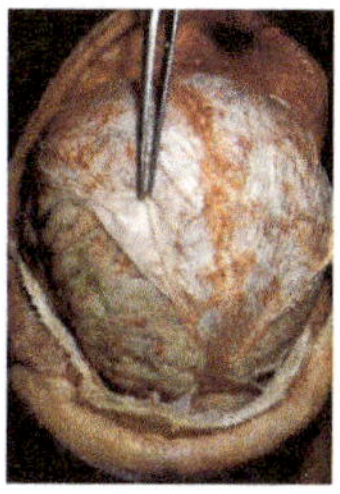

Acute infective meningitis

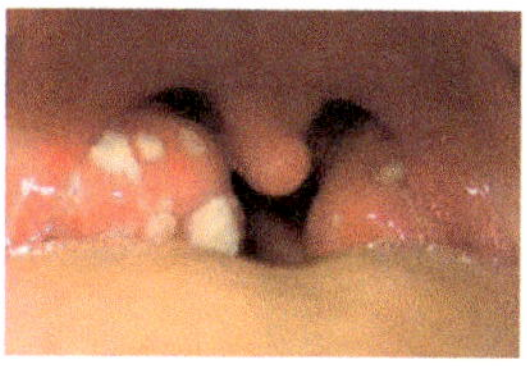

Acute tonsillitis

Diet and Inflammation

The Dietary Inflammatory Index (DII) is a score (number) that describes the potential of diet to modulate systemic inflammation within the body. As stated chronic inflammation is linked to most chronic diseases including arthritis, many types of cancer, cardiovascular diseases, inflammatory bowel diseases, and diabetes.

It has been known for many decades both that inflammation is linked to health and that diet is a major determinant of inflammation. Until the invention of the DII by scientists led by James R. Hébert at the Statewide South Carolina Cancer Prevention and Control Program in the University of South Carolina, no indicator of diet-related inflammation had ever been devised. The DII is unique among dietary indices in that it is based on results of studies published in the peer-reviewed literature and not any of the three methods typically used to create a dietary index; i.e., Basing it on 1) a particular cuisine or foodway (e.g., the Mediterranean, Macrobiotic or South Asian diet); 2) dietary guidelines (e.g., the Healthy Eating Index, which is based on the US Dietary Guidelines); or 3) results from a particular study (which reflect biases related to sample selection, response set biases such as social desirability). By contrast, the DII: 1) is grounded in peer-reviewed literature focusing specifically on inflammation (thus obviating idiosyncrasies of specific dietary assessment methods and limitations of exposure differences within populations); 2) can be adapted to virtually any dietary assessment method capable of providing estimates of nutrient intake; and 3) has been standardized to dietary intake from representative populations around the world, thus facilitating easy quantitative comparisons across studies.

Since its invention in 2004 and the publication of a now-defunct earlier-version of the DII in December 2009, the DII went through a major overhaul, resulting in a new version that replaced the old version, published first on-line in 2013 and then in hard copy in 2014. This new version is superior to the earlier one in a number of ways: 1) it is based on a larger, more robust literature of 1,943 (vs. 927) articles that were reviewed and scored; 2) creation of a global dataset based on intake measures from populations in 11 countries around the world, thus allowing comparison of results from studies conducted anywhere in the world; and 3) scoring such that lower, more negative, scores indicate anti-inflammation, while higher, more positive, scores are more pro-inflammatory.

This new, improved version of the DII has been subjected to construct validation, which tested (and subsequently confirmed) its ability to predict blood levels of inflammatory markers. The first of these tests showed the DII could predict repeat measures of c-reactive protein (CRP) from the Seasonal Variation of Blood Cholesterol, an intensive follow-up study of 559 adult men and women conducted in Massachusetts. The second, based on data from 2,567 women across the USA participating in the Women's Health Initiative Observational Study from 1993–1998, showed the DII's ability to predict levels of interleukin (IL)-6 and tumor necrosis factor-alpha receptor-2 (TNFα-R2) and a combined inflammatory biomarker score (consisting of IL-6, TNFα-R2, and CRP). Subsequently, the DII has been shown to have positive associations with IL-6 and homocysteine in the Asklepios Study in Belgium, CRP among police officers in Buffalo, NY, USA and inversely correlated with SNP rs2243250 in IL-4 among controls in the Bellvitge Colorectal Cancer Study in Spain.

Derivation and Computation

Briefly, based on a search of the literature from 1950 to the end of 2010, 45 food parameters were identified among foods, nutrients, and other food components that were associated with 6 plasma inflammatory markers (IL-1β, IL-4, IL-6, IL-10, TNF-α and CRP). A specific article inflammatory effect score for each food parameter on the basis of the literature review and taking into account the quality and number of published papers (1,943 articles were reviewed and scored). For each study participant in a study, the dietary data is first linked to a global database that was developed based on 11 datasets from around the world (US – NHANES; UK – The National Diet & Nutrition Survey; Bahrain – National Nutrition Survey for Adult Bahrainis; Mexico – Mexican National Health and Nutrition Survey; Australia – National Nutrition Survey; South Korea – KNHANES; Taiwan – Nutrition and Health Survey in Taiwan; India – Indian Diet Study; New Zealand – National Nutrition Survey) and thus provides a robust estimate of the mean and the standard deviation of these 45 parameters.[2] Each subject's exposure relative to the "standard global mean" is expressed as a z-score that is derived by subtracting the "standard global mean" from the amount reported, and dividing this value by its standard deviation. To minimize the effect of "right skewing", this value was then converted to a centered percentile score. The subject's DII score was computed by multiplying these values by the specific article inflammatory effect score for each food parameter and then summing together all these 45 values according to the following formula, $DII=b_1*n_1+b_2*n_2..........b_{45}*n_{45}$, where b_i refers to the literature-derived inflammatory effect score for each of the evaluated food parameter and n_i refers to the food parameter-specific centered percentile, which were derived from the dietary data, per each i from 1 to 45.

Accuracy

The DII is uniquely and strongly based on empirical evidence available in the peer-reviewed literature on the relationships between dietary factors and important inflammatory markers. It is important to note, however, that, as an index that superimposes on a method of dietary assessment, the DII is dependent on the accuracy of the dietary assessment method used. The DII cannot make up for deficiencies/ inaccuracies in measuring dietary intake.

Disease Prevention and Causation

Besides studies focusing on markers of inflammation in blood, the DII has been associated with a large number of actual health outcomes including:

- components of the metabolic syndrome, in a Spanish cohort and among US police officers;
- asthma and lung function in Australia;
- lung cancer and other respiratory conditions in Italy;
- esophageal cancer in Sweden, Italy, and Iran;
- colorectal cancer, in two populations of US women, Italian men and women, men and women in the National Institutes of Health-American Association of Retired Persons Diet and Health Study and a case-control study in Spain;
- female breast cancer in Germany and Sweden;
- prostate cancer, in Italy and Jamaica;
- pancreatic cancer in Italy;
- cardiovascular diseases, in the PREvencio´n con DIeta MEDiterra´nea (PREDIMED) Trial and the Seguimiento Universidad de Navarra (SUN) cohort in Spain, and a follow-up study of Australian men;
- depression in Spain;
- telomere length (an indicator of aging on a DNA level) in the Spanish PREDIMED Trial;
- overall mortality in American and Swedish women; and
- bone mineral density in Iran.

Other Factors That Can Influence Inflammation

Besides dietary factors, physical activity, fitness, sleep, shift work, and stress can affect inflammation. Also, there are auto-immune and other conditions that can influence inflammation. It has been shown that these other factors also may be related to the DII.

Advantages and Disadvantages of the DII

Advantages of the DII over other indices include that it: 1) focuses on a particular and very important mechanism of how dietary components affect health through inflammation; 2) is grounded in peer-reviewed literature focusing specifically on inflammatory markers known to affect health well-being; 3) can be adapted to virtually any dietary assessment method that provides estimates of nutrient intake; and 4) is standardized to dietary intake from representative populations around the world, thus facilitating easy quantitative comparisons across studies.

Disadvantages include that: 1) it is dependent on the quality of the dietary assessment upon which the computation is based (it cannot make up for deficiencies in the methods of obtaining the dietary data); and 2) it is not focused specifically on other effects of diet, though it is correlated (r (correlation coefficient) around $|0.50|$) with other diet indices that purport to assess diet quality.

Criticism and Alternatives

Criticisms include that the DII is not up to date. It must be noted that though the index was refined by the inclusion of three more years (from 2008 through 2010) of publications and more than doubling of the literature base, no major change in the overall thrust of the literature base was evident.

Exercise and Inflammation

Exercise-induced Acute Inflammation

Acute inflammation of the muscle cells, as understood in exercise physiology, can result after induced eccentric and concentric muscle training. Participation in eccentric training and conditioning, including resistance training and activities that emphasize eccentric lengthening of the muscle including downhill running on a moderate to high incline can result in considerable soreness within 24 to 48 hours, even though blood lactate levels, previously thought to cause muscle soreness, were much higher with level running. This delayed onset muscle soreness (DOMS) results from structural damage to the contractile filaments and z-disks, which has been noted especially in marathon runners whose muscle fibers revealed remarkable damage to the muscle fibers after both training and marathon competition. The onset and timing of this gradient damage to the muscle parallels the degree of muscle soreness experienced by the runners.

Z-disks are the point of contact for the contractile proteins. They provide structural support for transmission of force when muscle fibers are activated to shorten. However, in marathon runners and those who subscribe to the overload principle to enhance their muscles, show moderate Z-disk streaming and major disruption of thick and thin filaments in parallel groups of sarcomeres as a result of the force of eccentric actions or stretching of tightened muscle fibers.

This disruption of muscle fibers triggers white blood cells to increase following induced muscle soreness, leading to the inflammatory response observation from induced muscle soreness. Elevations in plasma enzymes, myoglobinemia, and abnormal muscle histology and ultrastructure are concluded to be associated with inflammatory response. High tension in the contractile-elastic system of muscle results in structural damage to the muscle fiber and plasmalemma and its epimysium, perimysium, and/or endomysium. The mysium damage disrupts calcium homeostasis in injured fibers and fiber bundles, resulting in necrosis that peaks about 48 hours after exercise. The products of macrophage activity and intracellular contents (such as histamines, kinins, and K^+) accumulate outside cells. These substances then stimulate free nerve endings in the muscle; a process that appears accentuated by eccentric exercise, in which large forces are distributed over a relatively small cross-sectional area of the muscle.

Post-inflammatory Muscle Growth and Repair

There is a known relationship between inflammation and muscle growth. For instance, high doses of anti-inflammatory medicines (e.g., NSAIDs) are able to blunt muscle growth. Cold therapy has been shown to negatively affect muscle growth as well. Reducing inflammation results in decreased macrophage activity and lower levels of IGF-1 Acute effects of cold therapy on training adaptations show reduced satellite cell proliferation. Long term effects include less muscular hypertrophy and an altered cell structure of muscle fibers.

It has been further theorized that the acute localized inflammatory responses to muscular contraction during exercise, as described above, are a necessary precursor to muscle growth. As a response to muscular contractions, the acute inflammatory response initiates the breakdown and removal of damaged muscle tissue. Muscles can synthesize cytokines in response to contractions, such that the cytokines interleukin-1 beta (IL-1β), TNF-α, and IL-6 are expressed in skeletal muscle up to 5 days after exercise.

In particular, the increase in levels of IL-6 (interleukin 6), a myokine, can reach up to one hundred times that of resting levels. Depending on volume, intensity, and other training factors, the IL-6 increase associated with training initiates about 4 hours after resistance training and remains elevated for up to 24 hours.

These acute increases in cytokines, as a response to muscle contractions, help initiate the process of muscle repair and growth by activating satellite cells within the inflamed muscle. Satellite cells are crucial for skeletal muscle adaptation to exercise. They contribute to hypertrophy by providing new myonuclei and repair damaged segments of mature myofibers for successful regeneration following injury- or exercise-induced muscle damage; high-level powerlifters can have up to 100% more satellite cells than untrained controls.

A rapid and transient localization of the IL-6 receptor and increased IL-6 expression occurs in satellite cells following contractions. IL-6 has been shown to mediate hypertrophic muscle growth both *in vitro* and *in vivo*. Unaccustomed exercise can increase IL-6 by up to sixfold at 5 hours post-exercise and threefold 8 days after exercise. Also telling is the fact that NSAIDs can decrease satellite cell response to exercise, thereby reducing exercise-induced protein synthesis.

The increase in cytokines (myokines) after resistance exercise coincides with the decrease in levels of myostatin, a protein that inhibits muscle differentiation and growth. The cytokine response to resistance exercise and moderate-intensity running occur differently, with the latter causing a more prolonged response, especially at the 12–24 hour mark.

Developing research has demonstrated that many of the benefits of exercise are mediated through the role of skeletal muscle as an endocrine organ. That is, contracting muscles release multiple substances known as myokines, including but not limited to those cited in the above description, which promote the growth of new tissue, tissue repair, and various anti-inflammatory functions, which in turn reduce the risk of developing various inflammatory diseases. The new view that muscle is an endocrine organ is transforming our understanding of exercise physiology and with it, of the role of inflammation in adaptation to stress.

Chronic Inflammation and Muscle Loss

Both chronic and extreme inflammation are associated with disruptions of anabolic signals initiating muscle growth. Chronic inflammation has been implicated as part of the cause of the muscle loss that occurs with aging. Increased protein levels of myostatin have been described in patients with diseases characterized by chronic low-grade inflammation. Increased levels of TNF-α can suppress the AKT/mTOR pathway, a crucial pathway for regulating skeletal muscle hypertrophy, thereby increasing muscle catabolism. Cytokines may antagonize the anabolic effects of insulin-like growth factor 1 (IGF-1). In the case of sepsis, an extreme whole body inflammatory state, the synthesis of both myofibrillar and sarcoplasmic proteins are inhibited, with the inhibition taking place preferentially in fast-twitch muscle fibers. Sepsis is also able to prevent leucine from stimulating muscle protein synthesis. In animal models, when inflammation is created, mTOR loses its ability to be stimulated by muscle growth.

Exercise as a Treatment for Inflammation

Regular physical activity is reported to decrease markers of inflammation, although the correlation is imperfect and seems to reveal differing results contingent upon training intensity. For instance, while baseline measurements of circulating inflammatory markers do not seem to differ greatly between healthy trained and untrained adults, long-term training may help reduce chronic low-grade inflammation. On the other hand, levels of the anti-inflammatory myokine IL-6 (interleukin 6) remained elevated longer into the recovery period following an acute bout of exercise in patients with inflammatory diseases, relative to the recovery of healthy controls. It may well be that low-intensity training can reduce resting pro-inflammatory markers (CRP, IL-6), while moderate-intensity training has milder and less-established anti-inflammatory benefits. There is a strong relationship between exhaustive exercise and chronic low-grade inflammation. Marathon running may enhance IL-6 levels as much as 100 times over normal and increases total leuckocyte count and neturophil mobilization.

Regarding the above, IL-6 had previously been classified as a proinflammatory cytokine. Therefore, it was first thought that the exercise-induced IL-6 response was related to muscle damage. However, it has become evident that eccentric exercise is not associated with a larger increase in plasma IL-6 than exercise involving concentric "nondamaging" muscle contractions. This finding clearly demonstrates that muscle damage is not required to provoke an increase in plasma IL-6 during exercise. As a matter of fact, eccentric exercise may result in a delayed peak and a much slower decrease of plasma IL-6 during recovery.

Recent work has shown that both upstream and downstream signalling pathways for IL-6 differ markedly between myocytes and macrophages. It appears that unlike IL-6 signalling in macrophages, which is dependent upon activation of the NFκB signalling pathway, intramuscular IL-6 expression is regulated by a network of signalling cascades, including the Ca2+/NFAT and glycogen/p38 MAPK pathways. Thus, when IL-6 is signalling in monocytes or macrophages, it creates a pro-inflammatory response, whereas IL-6 activation and signalling in muscle is totally independent of a preceding TNF-response or NFκB activation, and is anti-inflammatory.

Several studies show that markers of inflammation are reduced following longer-term behavioural changes involving both reduced energy intake and a regular program of increased physical activity, and that, in particular, IL-6 was miscast as an inflammatory marker. For example, the anti-inflammatory effects of IL-6 have been demonstrated by IL-6 stimulating the production of the classical anti-inflammatory cytokines IL-1ra and IL-10. As such, individuals pursuing exercise as a means to treat the causal factors underlying chronic inflammation are pursuing a course of action strongly supported by current research, as an inactive lifestyle is strongly associated with the development and progression of multiple inflammatory diseases. Note that cautions regarding over-exertion may apply in certain cases, as discussed above, though this concern rarely applies to the general population.

Signal-to-noise Theory

Given that localized acute inflammation is a necessary component for muscle growth, and that chronic low-grade inflammation is associated with a disruption of anabolic signals initiating muscle growth, it has been theorized that a signal-to-noise model may best describe the relationship between inflammation and muscle growth. By keeping the "noise" of chronic inflammation to a minimum, the localized acute inflammatory response signals a stronger anabolic response than could be achieved with higher levels of chronic inflammation.

Appendicitis

Appendicitis is inflammation of the appendix. Symptoms commonly include right lower abdominal pain, nausea, vomiting, and decreased appetite. However, approximately 40% of people do not have these typical symptoms. Severe complications of a ruptured appendix include widespread, painful inflammation of the inner lining of the abdominal wall and sepsis.

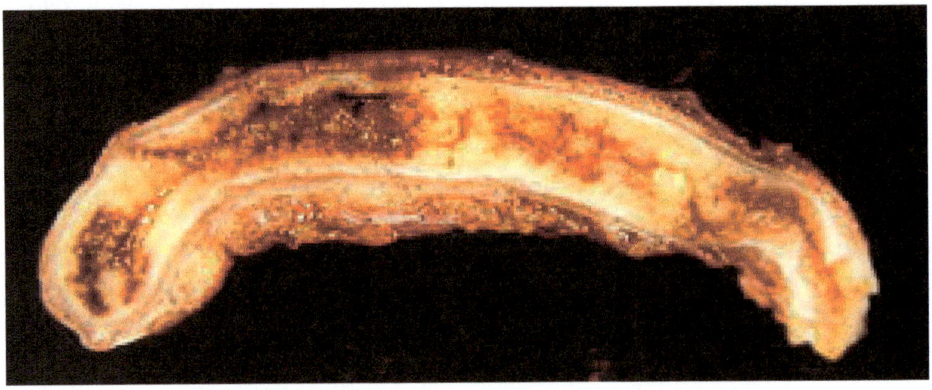

An acutely inflamed and enlarged appendix, sliced lengthwise.

Appendicitis is caused by a blockage of the hollow portion of the appendix. This is most commonly due to a calcified "stone" made of feces. Inflamed lymphoid tissue from a viral infection, parasites, gallstone, or tumors may also cause the blockage. This blockage leads to increased pressures in the appendix, decreased blood flow to the tissues of the appendix, and bacterial growth inside the appendix causing inflammation. The combination of inflammation, reduced blood flow to the appendix and distention of the appendix causes tissue injury and tissue death. If this process is left untreated, the appendix may burst, releasing bacteria into the abdominal cavity, leading to severe abdominal pain and increased complications.

The diagnosis of appendicitis is largely based on the person's signs and symptoms. In cases where the diagnosis cannot be made based on the person's history and physical exam, close observation, radiographic imaging and laboratory tests can be helpful. The two most common imaging tests used are an ultrasound and computed tomography (CT scan). CT scan has been shown to be more accurate than ultrasound in detecting acute appendicitis. However, ultrasound may be preferred as the first imaging test in children and pregnant women because of the risks associated with radiation exposure from CT scans.

The standard treatment for acute appendicitis is surgical removal of the appendix. This may be done by an open incision in the abdomen (laparotomy) or through a few smaller incisions with the help of cameras (laparoscopy). Surgery decreases the risk of side effects or death associated with rupture of the appendix. Antibiotics may be equally effective in certain cases of non-ruptured appendicitis. It is one of the most common and significant causes of severe abdominal pain that comes on quickly worldwide. In 2013 about 16 million cases of appendicitis occurred. This resulted in 72,000 deaths globally. In the United States, appendicitis is the most common cause of acute abdominal pain requiring surgery. Each year in the United States, more than 300,000 people with appendicitis have their appendix surgically removed. Reginald Fitz is credited with being the first person to describe the condition in 1886.

Signs and Symptoms

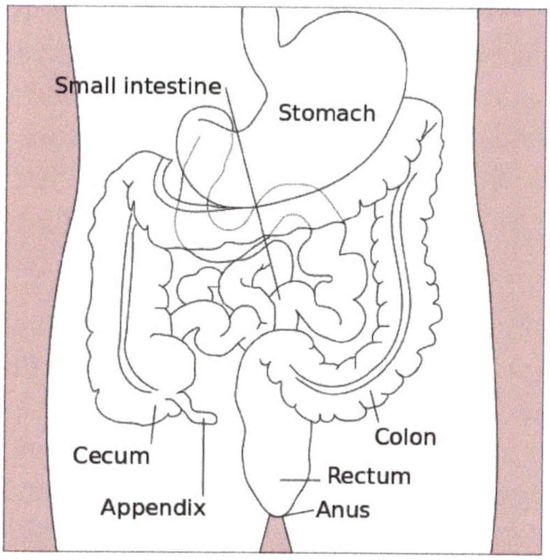

Location of the appendix in the digestive system

The presentation of acute appendicitis includes abdominal pain, nausea, vomiting, and fever. As the appendix becomes more swollen and inflamed, it begins to irritate the adjoining abdominal wall. This leads to the localization of the pain to the right lower quadrant. This classic migration of pain may not be seen in children under three years. This pain can be elicited through signs and can be severe. Signs include localized findings in the right iliac fossa. The abdominal wall becomes very sensitive to gentle pressure (palpation). There is severe pain on sudden release of deep pressure in the lower abdomen (rebound tenderness). If the appendix is retrocecal (localized behind the cecum), even deep pressure in the right lower quadrant may fail to elicit tenderness (silent appendix). This is because the cecum, distended with gas, protects the inflamed appendix from pressure. Similarly, if the appendix lies entirely within the pelvis, there is usually complete absence of abdominal rigidity. In such cases, a digital rectal examination elicits tenderness in the rectovesical pouch. Coughing causes point tenderness in this area (McBurney's point).

Causes

Acute appendicitis seems to be the end result of a primary obstruction of the appendix. Once this obstruction occurs, the appendix becomes filled with mucus and swells. This continued production of mucus leads to increased pressures within the lumen and the walls of the appendix. The increased pressure results in thrombosis and occlusion of the small vessels, and stasis of lymphatic flow. At this point spontaneous recovery rarely occurs. As the occlusion of blood vessels progresses, the appendix becomes ischemic and then necrotic. As bacteria begin to leak out through the dying walls, pus forms within and around the appendix (suppuration). The end result is appendiceal rupture (a 'burst appendix') causing peritonitis, which may lead to sepsis and eventually death. These events are responsible for the slowly evolving abdominal pain and other commonly associated symptoms.

The causative agents include bezoars, foreign bodies, trauma, intestinal worms, lymphadenitis and, most commonly, calcified fecal deposits that are known as appendicoliths or fecaliths. The occurrence of obstructing fecaliths has attracted attention since their presence in people with appendicitis is higher in developed than in developing countries. In addition an appendiceal fecalith is commonly associated with complicated appendicitis. Fecal stasis and arrest may play a role, as demonstrated by people with acute appendicitis having fewer bowel movements per week compared with healthy controls.

The occurrence of a fecalith in the appendix was thought to be attributed to a right-sided fecal retention reservoir in the colon and a prolonged transit time. However, a prolonged transit time was not observed in subsequent studies. From epidemiological data, it has been stated that diverticular disease and adenomatous polyps were unknown and colon cancer exceedingly rare in communities exempt from appendicitis. And acute appendicitis has been shown to occur antecedent to cancer in the colon and rectum. Several studies offer evidence that a low fiber intake is involved in the pathogenesis of appendicitis. This low intake of dietary fiber is in accordance with the occurrence of a right-sided fecal reservoir and the fact that dietary fiber reduces transit time.

Diagnosis

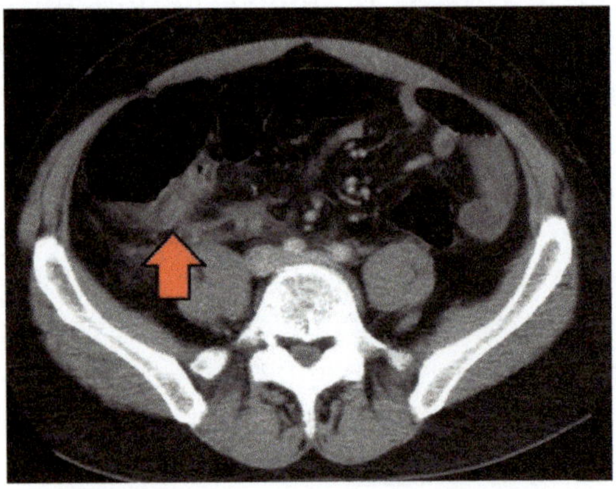

Appendicitis as seen on CT imaging

Diagnosis is based on a medical history (symptoms) and physical examination which can be supported by an elevation of neutrophilic white blood cells and imaging studies if needed. (Neutrophils are the primary white blood cells that respond to a bacterial infection.) Histories fall into two categories, typical and atypical.

Typical appendicitis includes several hours of generalized abdominal pain that begins in the region of the umbilicus with associated anorexia, nausea, or vomiting. The pain then "localizes" into the right lower quadrant where the tenderness increases in intensity. It is possible the pain could localize to the left lower quadrant in people with situs inversus totalis. The combination of pain, anorexia, leukocytosis, and fever is classic.

Atypical histories lack this typical progression and may include pain in the right lower quadrant as an initial symptom. Irritation of the peritoneum (inside lining of the abdominal wall) can lead to increased pain on movement, or jolting, for example going over speedbumps. Atypical histories often require imaging with ultrasound and/or CT scanning.

Clinical

- Aure-Rozanova's sign: Increased pain on palpation with finger in right Petit triangle (can be a positive Shchetkin-Bloomberg's).
- Bartomier-Michelson's sign: Increased pain on palpation at the right iliac region as the person being examined lies on his or her left side compared to when he/she lies on the back.
- Dunphy's sign: Increased pain in the right lower quadrant with coughing.
- Hamburger sign: The patient refuses to eat (anorexia is 80% specific for appendicitis)
- Kocher's (Kosher's) sign: From the person's medical history, the start of pain in the umbilical region with a subsequent shift to the right iliac region.
- Massouh sign: Developed in and popular in southwest England, the examiner performs a firm swish with his or her index and middle finger across the abdomen from the xiphoid process to the left and the right iliac fossa. A positive Massouh sign is a grimace of the person being examined upon a right sided (and not left) sweep.
- Obturator sign: The person being evaluated lies on her or his back with the hip and knee both flexed at ninety degrees. The examiner holds the person's ankle with one hand and knee with the other hand. The examiner rotates the hip by moving the person's ankle away from his or her body while allowing the knee to move only inward. A positive test is pain with internal rotation of the hip.
- Psoas sign, also known as "Obraztsova's sign", is right lower-quadrant pain

that is produced with either the passive extension of the right hip or by the active flexion of the person's right hip while supine. The pain that is elicited is due to inflammation of the peritoneum overlying the iliopsoas muscles and inflammation of the psoas muscles themselves. Straightening out the leg causes pain because it stretches these muscles, while flexing the hip activates the iliopsoas and causes pain.

- Rovsing's sign: Pain in the lower right abdominal quadrant with continuous deep palpation starting from the left iliac fossa upwards (counterclockwise along the colon). The thought is there will be increased pressure around the appendix by pushing bowel contents and air toward the ileocaecal valve provoking right-sided abdominal pain.
- Sitkovskiy (Rosenstein)'s sign: Increased pain in the right iliac region as the person is being examined lies on his/her left side.

Blood and Urine Test

While there is no laboratory test specific for appendicitis, a complete blood count (CBC) is done to check for signs of infection. Although 70–90 percent of people with appendicitis may have an elevated white blood cell (WBC) count, there are many other abdominal and pelvic conditions that can cause the WBC count to be elevated. Due to its low sensitivity and specificity, on its own, WBC is not seen as a good indicator of appendicitis.

A urinalysis generally does not show infection, but it is important for determining pregnancy status, especially the possibility of an ectopic pregnancy in women of childbearing age. The urinalysis is also important for ruling out a urinary tract infection as the cause of abdominal pain. The presence of more than 20 WBC per high-power field in the urine is more suggestive of a urinary tract disorder.

Imaging

In children the clinical examination is important to determine which children with abdominal pain should receive immediate surgical consultation and which should receive diagnostic imaging. Because of the health risks of exposing children to radiation, ultrasound is the preferred first choice with CT scan being a legitimate follow-up if the ultrasound is inconclusive. CT scan is more accurate than ultrasound for the diagnosis of appendicitis in adults and adolescents. CT scan has a sensitivity of 94%, specificity of 95%. Ultrasonography had an overall sensitivity of 86%, a specificity of 81%.

Ultrasound

Ultrasonography and Doppler sonography are useful to detect appendicitis, especially in children. Ultrasound can show free fluid collection in the right iliac fossa, along with a visible appendix with increased blood flow when using color Doppler, and noncompressibility of the appendix, as it is essentially a walled off abscess. Other secondary sonographic signs of acute appendicitis include the presence of echogenic mesenteric fat surrounding the appendix and the acoustic shadowing of an appendicolith. In some cases (approximately 5%), ultrasonography of the iliac fossa does not reveal any abnormalities despite the presence of appendicitis. This false negative finding is especially true of early appendicitis before the appendix has become significantly distended. In addition, false negative findings are more common in adults where larger amounts of fat and bowel gas make visualizing the appendix technically difficult. Despite these limitations, sonographic imaging in experienced hands can often distinguish between appendicitis and other diseases with similar symptoms. Some of these conditions include inflammation of lymph nodes near the appendix or pain originating from other pelvic organs such as the ovaries or Fallopian tubes.

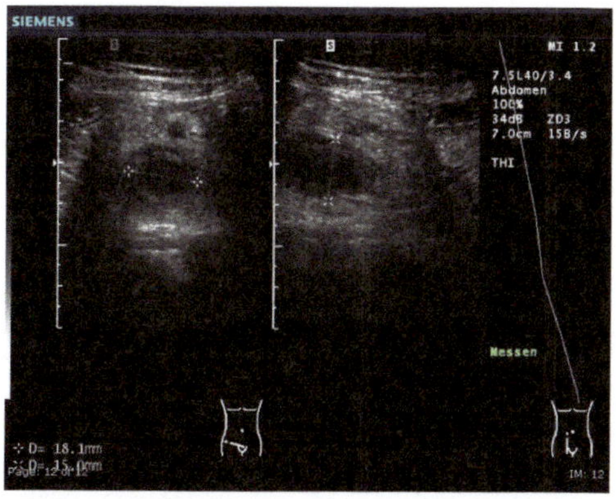

Ultrasound image of acute appendicitis

Computed Tomography

Where it is readily available, computed tomography (CT) has become frequently used, especially in people whose diagnosis is not obvious on history and physical examination. Concerns about radiation tend to limit use of CT in pregnant women and children, especially with the increasingly widespread usage of MRI.

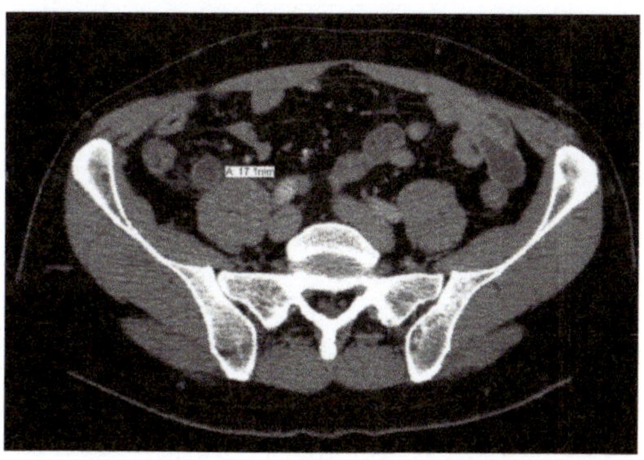
A CT scan demonstrating acute appendicitis (note the appendix has a diameter of 17.1 mm and there is surrounding fat stranding)

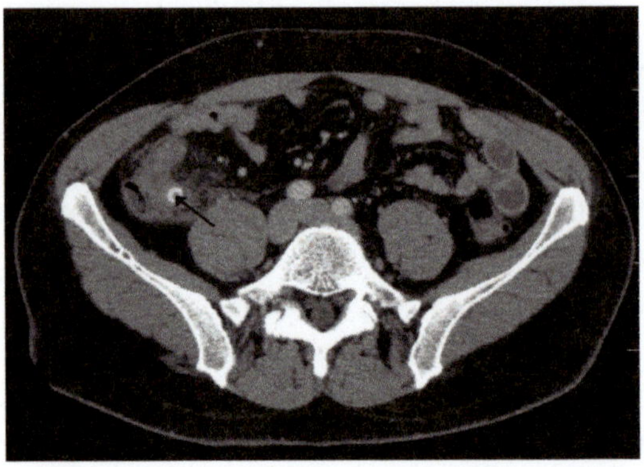

A fecalith marked by the arrow that has resulted in acute appendicitis.

The accurate diagnosis of appendicitis is multi-tiered, with the size of the appendix having the strongest positive predictive value, while indirect features can either increase or decrease sensitivity and specificity. A size of over 6 mm is both 95% sensitive and specific for appendicitis.

However, because the appendix can be filled with fecal material, causing intraluminal distention, this criterion has shown limited utility in more recent meta analyses. This is as opposed to ultrasound, in which the wall of the appendix can be more easily distinguished from intraluminal feces. In such scenarios, ancillary features such as increased wall enhancement as compared to adjacent bowel and inflammation of the surrounding fat, or fat stranding, can be supportive of the diagnosis, although their absence does not preclude it. In severe cases with perforation, an adjacent phlegmon or abscess can be seen. Dense fluid layering in the pelvis can also result, related to either pus or enteric spillage. When patients are thin or younger, the relative absence of fat can make the appendix and surrounding fat stranding difficult to see.

Magnetic Resonance Imaging

MRI use has become increasingly common for diagnosis of appendicitis in children and pregnant patients due to the radiation dosage that, while of nearly negligible risk in healthy adults, can be harmful to children or the developing fetus. In pregnancy, it has been found to be more useful during the second and third trimester, particularly as the enlargening uterus displaces the appendix, making it difficult to find by ultrasound. The periappendiceal stranding that is reflected on CT by fat stranding on MRI appears as increased fluid signal on T2 weighted sequences. First trimester pregnancies are usually not candidates for MRI, as the fetus is still undergoing organogenesis, and there are no long-term studies to date regarding its potential risks or side effects.

X-ray

In general, plain abdominal radiography (PAR) is not useful in making the diagnosis of appendicitis and should not be routinely obtained from a person being evaluated for appendicitis. Plain abdominal films may be useful for the detection of ureteral calculi, small bowel obstruction, or perforated ulcer, but these conditions are rarely confused with appendicitis. An opaque fecalith can be identified in the right lower quadrant in fewer than 5% of people being evaluated for appendicitis. A barium enema has proven to be a poor diagnostic tool for appendicitis. While failure of the appendix to fill during a barium enema has been associated with appendicitis, up to 20% of normal appendices do not fill.

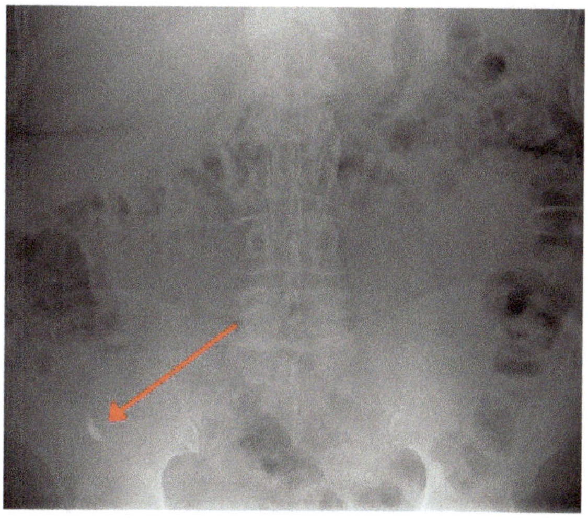

Appendicolith as seen on plain X-ray

Scoring Systems

Alvarado score	
Migratory right iliac fossa pain	1 point
Anorexia	1 point
Nausea and vomiting	1 point
Right iliac fossa tenderness	2 points
Rebound abdominal tenderness	1 point
Fever	1 point
High white blood cell count (leukocytosis)	2 points
Shift to left (segmented neutrophils)	1 point
Total score	**10 points**

No excellent scoring system exists to determine if a child has appendicitis. The Alvarado score and pediatric appendicitis score are useful but not definitive.

The Alvarado score is the most widely used scoring system. A score below 5 suggests against a diagnosis of appendicitis, whereas a score of 7 or more is predictive of acute appendicitis. In a person with an equivocal score of 5 or 6, a CT scan or ultrasound exam may be used to reduce the rate of negative appendectomy.

Pathology

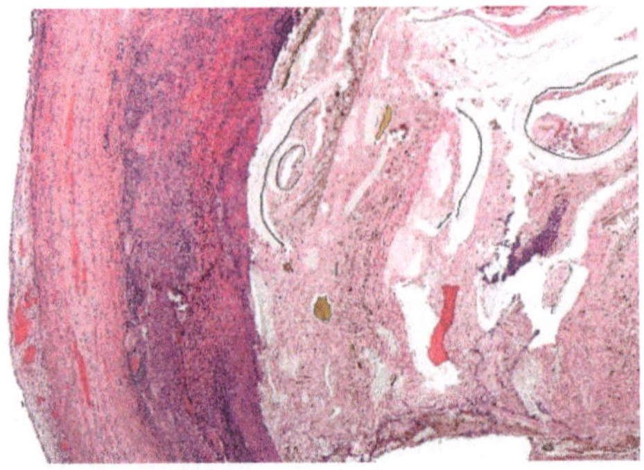

Micrograph of appendicitis and periappendicitis. H&E stain.

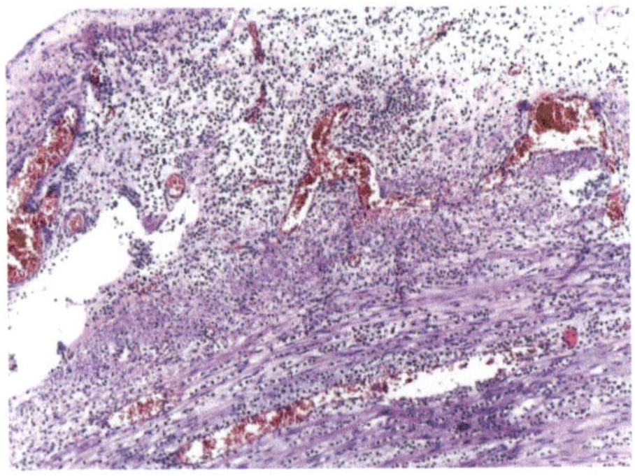

Micrograph of appendicitis showing neutrophils in the muscularis propria. H&E stain.

The definitive diagnosis is based on pathology. The histologic finding of appendicitis is neutrophilic infiltrate of the muscularis propria.

Periappendicits, inflammation of tissues around the appendix, is often found in conjunction with other abdominal pathology.

Differential Diagnosis

Children: Gastroenteritis, mesenteric adenitis, Meckel's diverticulitis, intussusception, Henoch–Schönlein purpura, lobar pneumonia, urinary tract infection (abdominal pain in the absence of other symptoms can occur in children with UTI), new-onset Crohn's disease or ulcerative colitis, pancreatitis, and abdominal trauma from child abuse; distal intestinal obstruction syndrome in children with cystic fibrosis; typhlitis in children with leukemia.

Women: A pregnancy test is important for all women of childbearing age since an ectopic pregnancy can have signs and symptoms similar to those of appendicitis. Other obstetrical/gynecological causes of similar abdominal pain in women include pelvic inflammatory disease, ovarian torsion, menarche, dysmenorrhea, endometriosis, and Mittelschmerz (the passing of an egg in the ovaries approximately two weeks before menstruation).

Men: testicular torsion

Adults: new-onset Crohn's disease, ulcerative colitis, regional enteritis, renal colic, perforated peptic ulcer, pancreatitis, rectus sheath hematoma and epiploic appendagitis.

Elderly: diverticulitis, intestinal obstruction, colonic carcinoma, mesenteric ischemia, leaking aortic aneurysm.

The term "pseudoappendicitis" is used to describe a condition mimicking appendicitis. It can be associated with *Yersinia enterocolitica*.

Management

Acute appendicitis is typically managed by surgery. However, in uncomplicated cases, antibiotics are effective and safe. While antibiotics are effective for treating uncomplicated appendicitis, 26% of people had a recurrence within a year and required eventual appendectomy.

In people with inflammatory bowel disease such as Crohn's disease or ulcerative colitis who present with appendicitis, surgical intervention is contraindicated, as the normal healing response following surgery is impaired by the underlying disease process, and the patients form non-healing fistulas, sinus tracts and enteric leakage. In such scenarios, the underlying disease process must be treated medically with DMARDs, as opposed to surgically.

Pain

Pain medications (such as morphine) do not appear to affect the accuracy of the clinical diagnosis of appendicitis and therefore should be given early in the patient's care. Historically there were concerns among some general surgeons that analgesics would affect the clinical exam in children, and some recommended that they not be given until the surgeon was able to examine the person.

Surgery

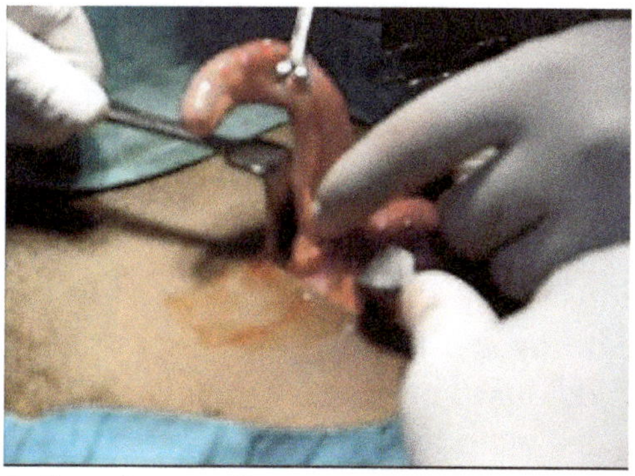

Inflamed appendix removal by open surgery

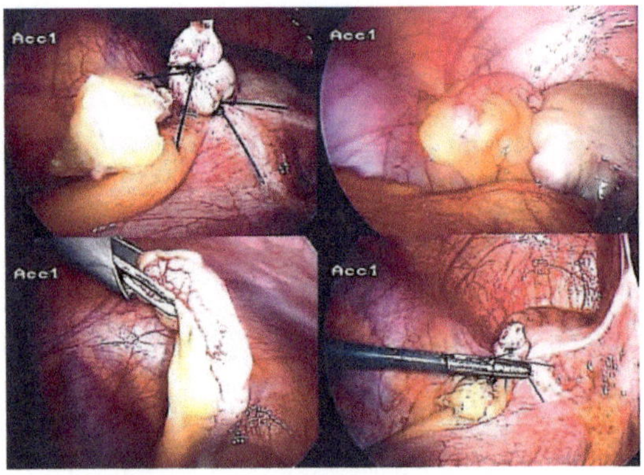

Laparoscopic appendectomy

The surgical procedure for the removal of the appendix is called an appendectomy. Appendectomy can be performed through open or laparoscopic surgery. Laparoscopic appendectomy has several advantages over open appendectomy as an intervention for acute appendicitis.

Open Appendectomy

For over a century, laparotomy (open appendectomy) was the standard treatment for acute appendicitis. This procedure consists of the removal of the infected appendix through a single large incision in the lower right area of the abdomen. The incision in a laparotomy is usually 2 to 3 inches (51 to 76 mm) long.

During an open appendectomy, the person with suspected appendicitis is placed under general anesthesia to keep the muscles completely relaxed and to keep the person unconscious. The incision is two to three inches (76 mm) long and it is made in the right lower abdomen, several inches above the hip bone. Once the incision opens the abdomen cavity and the appendix is identified, the surgeon removes the infected tissue and cuts the appendix from the surrounding tissue. After careful and close inspection of the infected area, and ensuring there are no signs that surrounding tissues are damaged or infected, the surgeon will start closing the incision. This means sewing the muscles and using surgical staples or stitches to close the skin up. To prevent infections, the incision is covered with a sterile bandage.

Laparoscopic Appendectomy

Laparoscopic appendectomy has become an increasingly prevalent intervention for acute appendicitis since its introduction in 1983. This surgical procedure consists of making three to four incisions in the abdomen, each 0.25 to 0.5 inches (6.4 to 12.7 mm) long. This type of appendectomy is made by inserting a special surgical tool called laparoscope into one of the incisions. The laparoscope is connected to a monitor outside the person's body and it is designed to help the surgeon to inspect the infected area in the abdomen. The other two incisions are made for the specific removal of the appendix by using surgical instruments. Laparoscopic surgery requires general anesthesia, and it can last up to two hours. Laparoscopic appendectomy has several advantages over open appendectomy, including a shorter post-operative recovery, less post-operative pain, and lower superficial surgical site infection rate. However, the occurrence of intra-abdominal abscess is almost three times more prevalent in laparoscopic appendectomy than open appendectomy.

Pre-surgery

The treatment begins by keeping the person who will be having surgery from eating or drinking for a given period, usually overnight. An intravenous drip is used to hydrate the person who will be having surgery. Antibiotics given intravenously such as cefuroxime and metronidazole may be administered early to help kill bacteria and thus reduce the spread of infection in the abdomen and postoperative complications in the abdomen or wound. Equivocal cases may become more difficult to assess with antibiotic treatment and benefit from serial examinations. If the stomach is empty (no food in the past six hours) general anaesthesia is usually used. Otherwise, spinal anaesthesia may be used.

Once the decision to perform an appendectomy has been made, the preparation procedure takes approximately one to two hours. Meanwhile, the surgeon will explain the surgery procedure and will present the risks that must be considered when performing an appendectomy. (With all surgeries there are risks that must be evaluated before performing the procedures.) The risks are different depending on the state of the appendix. If the appendix has not ruptured, the complication rate is only about 3% but if the appendix has ruptured, the complication rate rises to almost 59%. The most usual complications that can occur are pneumonia, hernia of the incision, thrombophlebitis, bleeding or adhesions. Recent evidence indicates that a delay in obtaining surgery after admission results in no measurable difference in outcomes to the person with appendicitis.

The surgeon will explain how long the recovery process should take. Abdomen hair is usually removed to avoid complications that may appear regarding the incision.

In most cases, patients going in for surgery experience nausea or vomiting that requires medication before surgery. Antibiotics along with pain medication may be administrated before appendectomies.

After Surgery

Hospital lengths of stay typically range from a few hours to a few days but can be a few weeks if complications occur. The recovery process may vary depending on the severity of the condition: if the appendix had ruptured or not before surgery. Appendix surgery recovery is generally a lot faster if the appendix did not rupture. It is important that people undergoing surgery respect their doctor's advice and limit their physical activity so the tissues can heal faster. Recovery after an appendectomy may not require diet changes or a lifestyle change.

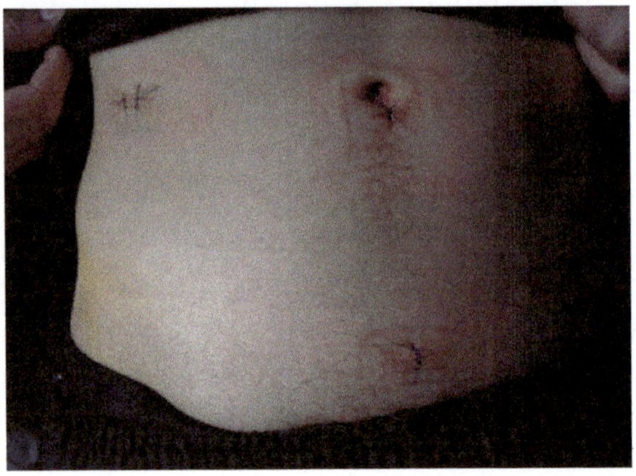

The stitches the day after having the appendix removed by laparoscopic surgery

Length of hospital stays for appendicitis varies on the severity of the condition. A study from the United States found that in 2010, the average appendicitis hospital stay was 1.8 days. For stays where the person's appendix had ruptured, the average length of stay was 5.2 days.

After surgery, the patient will be transferred to a postanesthesia care unit so his or her vital signs can be closely monitored to detect anesthesia- and/or surgery-related complications. Pain medication may be administered if necessary. After patients are completely awake, they are moved to a hospital room to recover. Most individuals will be offered clear liquids the day after the surgery, then progress to a regular diet when the intestines start to function properly. Patients are recommended to sit up on the edge of the bed and walk short distances several times a day. Moving is mandatory and pain medication may be given if necessary. Full recovery from appendectomies takes about four to six weeks but can be prolonged to up to eight weeks if the appendix had ruptured.

Prognosis

Most people with appendicitis recover easily after surgical treatment, but complications can occur if treatment is delayed or if peritonitis occurs. Recovery time depends on age, condition, complications, and other circumstances, including the amount of alcohol consumption, but usually is between 10 and 28 days. For young children (around 10 years old), the recovery takes three weeks.

The possibility of peritonitis is the reason why acute appendicitis warrants speedy evaluation and treatment. People with suspected appendicitis may have to undergo a medical evacuation. Appendectomies have occasionally been performed in emergency conditions (i.e., not in a proper hospital), when a timely medical evacuation was impossible.

Typical acute appendicitis responds quickly to appendectomy and occasionally will resolve spontaneously. If appendicitis resolves spontaneously, it remains controversial whether an elective interval appendectomy should be performed to prevent a recurrent episode of appendicitis. Atypical appendicitis (associated with suppurative appendicitis) is more difficult to diagnose and is more apt to be complicated even when operated early. In either condition, prompt diagnosis and appendectomy yield the best results with full recovery in two to four weeks usually. Mortality and severe complications are unusual but do occur, especially if peritonitis persists and is untreated.

Another entity known as appendicular lump is talked about. It happens when the appendix is not removed early during infection and omentum and intestine adhere to it, forming a palpable lump. During this period, surgery is risky unless there is pus formation evident by fever and toxicity or by USG. Medical management treats the condition.

An unusual complication of an appendectomy is "stump appendicitis": inflammation occurs in the remnant appendiceal stump left after a prior incomplete appendectomy. Stump appendicitis can occur months to years after initial appendectomy and can be identified with imaging modalities like ultrasound.

Epidemiology

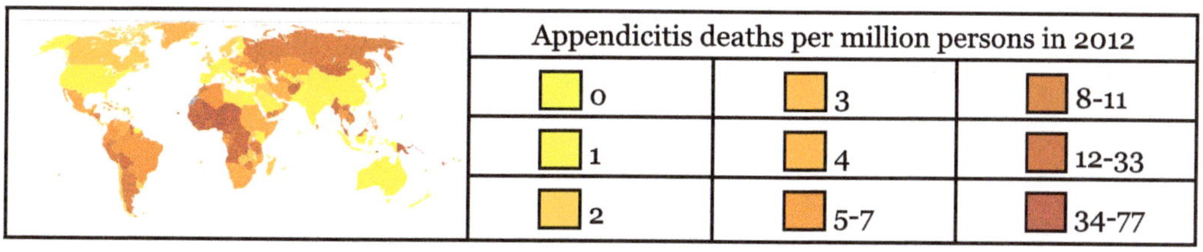

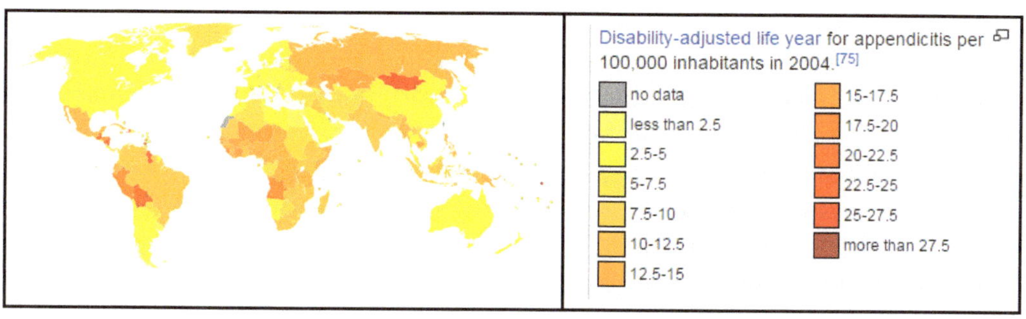

Appendicitis is most common between the ages of 5 and 40; the median age is 28. It tends to affect males, those in lower income groups and, for unknown reasons, people living in rural areas. In 2013 it resulted in 72,000 deaths globally down from 88,000 in 1990.

In the United States, there were nearly 293,000 hospitalizations involving appendicitis in 2010. Appendicitis is one of the most frequent diagnoses for emergency department visits resulting in hospitalization among children ages 5–17 years in the United States.

Bursitis

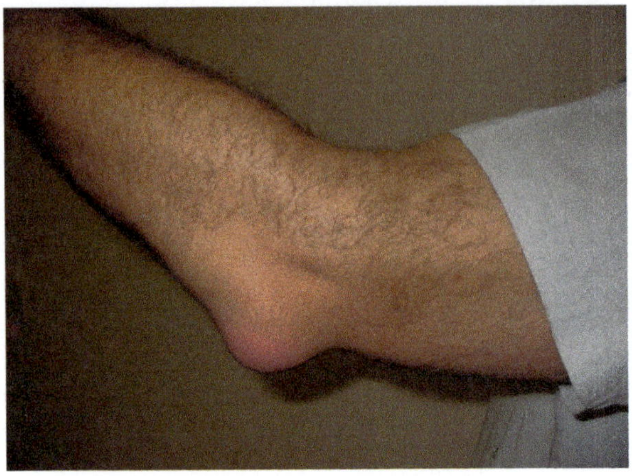

Example of elbow bursitis

Bursitis is the inflammation of one or more bursae (small sacs) of synovial fluid in the body. They are lined with a synovial membrane that secretes a lubricating synovial fluid. There are more than 150 bursae in the human body. The bursae rest at the points where internal functionaries, such as muscles and tendons, slide across bone. Healthy bursae create a smooth, almost frictionless functional gliding surface making normal movement painless. When bursitis occurs, however, movement relying on the inflamed bursa becomes difficult and painful. Moreover, movement of tendons and muscles over the inflamed bursa aggravates its inflammation, perpetuating the problem. Muscle can also be stiffened.

Signs and Symptoms

Bursitis commonly affects superficial bursae. These include the subacromial, prepatellar, retrocalcaneal, and pes anserinus bursae of the shoulder, knee, heel and shin, etc. Symptoms vary from localized warmth and erythema to joint pain and stiffness, to stinging pain that surrounds the joint around the inflamed bursa. In this condition, the pain usually is worse during and after activity, and then the bursa and the surrounding joint becomes stiff the next morning.

Cause

There can be several concurrent causes. Trauma, auto-immune disorders, infection and iatrogenic (medicine-related) factors can all cause bursitis. Bursitis is commonly caused by repetitive movement and excessive pressure. Shoulders, elbows and knees are the most commonly affected. Inflammation of the bursae may also be caused by other inflammatory conditions such as rheumatoid arthritis, scleroderma, systemic lupus erythematosus and gout. Immune deficiencies, including HIV and diabetes, can also cause bursitis. Infrequently, scoliosis can cause bursitis of the shoulders; however, shoulder bursitis is more commonly caused by overuse of the shoulder joint and related muscles.

Traumatic injury is another cause of bursitis. The inflammation irritates because the bursa no longer fits in the original small area between the bone and the functionary muscle or tendon. When the bone increases pressure upon the bursa, bursitis results. Sometimes the reason is unknown. It can also be associated with various other chronic systemic diseases.

Examples by Site

The most common examples of this condition:

- Prepatellar bursitis, “housemaid’s knee”
- Infrapatellar bursitis, “clergyman’s knee”
- Trochanteric bursitis, giving pain over lateral aspect of hip
- Olecranon bursitis, “student’s elbow”, characterised by pain and swelling in the elbow
- Subacromial bursitis, giving shoulder pain, is the most common form of bursitis.
- Achilles bursitis
- Retrocalcaneal bursitis
- Ischial bursitis, “weaver’s bottom”
- Iliopsoas bursitis
- Anserine bursitis

Treatment

It is important to differentiate between infected and non-infected bursitis. People may have surrounding cellulitis and systemic symptoms include a fever. The bursa should be aspirated to rule out an infectious process.

Bursae that are not infected can be treated symptomatically with rest, ice, elevation, physiotherapy, anti-inflammatory drugs and pain medication. Since bursitis is caused by increased friction from the adjacent structures, a compression bandage is not suggested because compression would create more friction around the joint. Chronic bursitis can be amenable to bursectomy and aspiration. Bursae that are infected require further investigation and antibiotic therapy. Steroid therapy may also be considered. In cases when all conservative treatment fails, surgical therapy may be necessary. In a bursectomy the bursa is cut out either endoscopically or with open surgery. The bursa grows back in place after a couple of weeks but without any inflammatory component.

Colitis

Colitis (pl. colitides) is an inflammation of the colon.

Colitis may be acute and self-limited or chronic, i.e. persistent, and broadly fits into the category of digestive diseases.

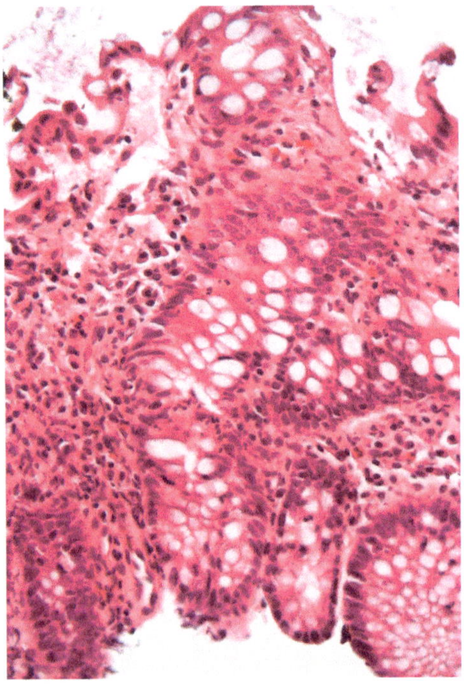

A micrograph demonstrating cryptitis, a microscopic correlate of colitis. H&E stain.

In a medical context, the label *colitis* (without qualification) is used if:

- The cause of the inflammation in the colon is undetermined; for example, *colitis* may be applied to *Crohn's disease* at a time when the diagnosis is unknown, or
- The context is clear; for example, an individual with ulcerative colitis is talking about their disease with a physician who knows the diagnosis.

Signs and Symptoms

The signs and symptoms of colitis are quite variable and dependent on the cause of the given colitis and factors that modify its course and severity.

Symptoms of colitis may include: mild to severe abdominal pain and tenderness (depending on the stage of the disease), recurring bloody diarrhea with/without pus in the stools, fecal incontinence, flatulence, fatigue, loss of appetite and unexplained weight loss.

More severe symptoms may include: shortness of breath, a fast or irregular heartbeat and fever.

Other less or rare non-specific symptoms that may accompany colitis include: arthritis, mouth ulcers, painful, red and swollen skin and irritated, red eyes.

Signs seen on colonoscopy include: colonic mucosal erythema (redness of the inner surface of the colon), ulcers, and bleeding.

Diagnosis

Symptoms suggestive of colitis are worked-up by obtaining the medical history, a physical examination and laboratory tests (CBC, electrolytes, stool culture and sensitivity, stool ova and parasites et cetera). Additional tests may include medical imaging (e.g. abdominal computed tomography, abdominal X-rays) and an examination with a camera inserted into the rectum (sigmoidoscopy, colonoscopy).

An important investigation in the assessment of colitis is biopsy. A very small piece of tissue (usually about 2mm) is removed from the bowel mucosa during endoscopy and examined under the microscope by a histopathologist. It can provide important information regarding the cause of the disease and the extent of bowel damage.

Types

There are many types of colitis. They are usually classified by the cause.

Types of colitis include:

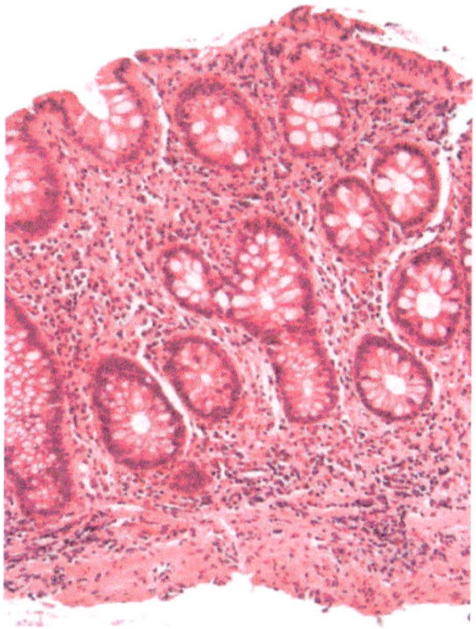

Micrograph showing intestinal crypt branching, a histopathological finding of chronic colitis. H&E stain.

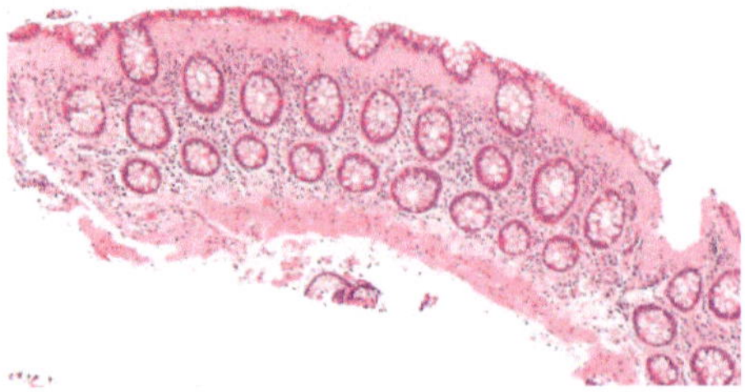

Micrograph of collagenous colitis. H&E stain.

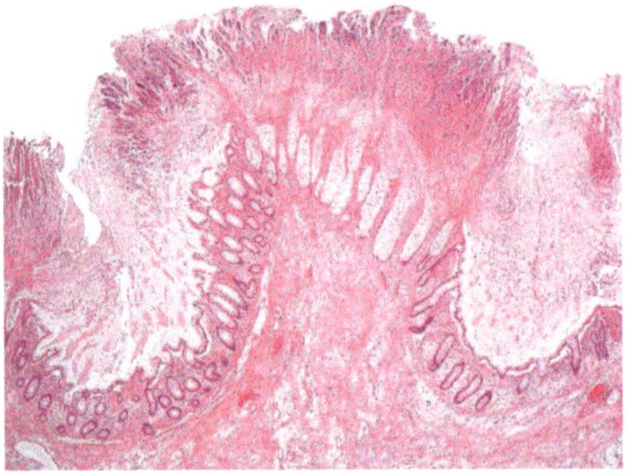

Micrograph of a colonic pseudomembrane, as may be seen in *Clostridium difficile* colitis, a type of infectious colitis.

Autoimmune

- Inflammatory bowel disease (IBD) – a group of chronic colitides.
  - Ulcerative colitis – a chronic colitis that affects the large intestine.
  - Crohn's disease – a type of IBD that often leads to colitis.

Idiopathic

- Microscopic colitis – a colitis is diagnosed by microscopic examination of colonic tissue; macroscopically it is normal appearing.
  - Lymphocytic colitis
  - Collagenous colitis

Iatrogenic

- Diversion colitis
- Chemical colitis

Vascular Disease

- Ischemic colitis

Infectious

- Infectious colitis

A well-known subtype of infectious colitis is *Clostridium difficile* colitis, which is informally abbreviated as "c diff colitis". It classically forms pseudomembranes and is often referred to as *pseudomembranous colitis*, which is its (non-specific) histomorphologic description.

Enterohemorrhagic colitis may be caused by Shiga toxin in *Shigella dysenteriae* or *Shigatoxigenic group* of *Escherichia coli* (STEC), which includes serotype O157:H7 and other enterohemorrhagic *E. coli*.

Parasitic infections, like those caused by *Entamoeba histolytica*, can also cause colitis.

Unclassifiable Colitides

Indeterminate colitis is the classification for colitis that has features of both *Crohn's disease* and *ulcerative colitis*. Indeterminate colitis' behaviour is usually closer to ulcerative colitis than Crohn's disease.

Atypical colitis is a phrase that is occasionally used by physicians for a colitis that does not conform to criteria for accepted types of colitis. It is not an accepted diagnosis *per se* and, as such, a colitis that cannot be definitively classified.

Treatment

Some people may be admitted into the hospital following the colonoscopy depending on results. It is sometimes necessary to get the patient started on a steroid to speed up the healing of the colon. It may also be necessary to get the patient hydrated from the fluid loss and iron replaced from the loss of blood. After a hospital stay, the patient may be put on a daily medication to manage their chronic colitis. The medication can be an anti-inflammatory or an immunosuppressant. There are many different types of medication used and the doctor will prescribe the one they see fit. If the patient doesn't respond, new medications will be tried until there is a good fit. Moreover, several studies recently have found significant relationship between colitis and dairy allergy (including: cow milk, cow milk UHT and casein) suggesting some patients may benefit from an elimination diet.

Antiviral Defense

These are the responses against viral infection and are mediated by cytokines and natural killer cells. Pathogens which are able to survive against inflammation and antiviral defense in turns enter into blood circulation. Blood contains another important component of innate immunity called complements. The pathogens are destroyed by typical classical and alternate pathways of the complement system. The innate immune responses many time fails to eradicate the pathogens. In those cases the immune system is evolved with more robust and powerful cells and antibodies of adaptive immune system.

Recognition System of Innate Immunity

Innate immune system recognizes the structures present on the microbial pathogens and are collectively called pathogen associated molecular pattern (PAMP). Similarly innate immune system also recognizes the molecules produced by the damaged cell and are collectively called damage associated molecular pattern (DAMP). The PAMP and DAMP are collectively called pattern recognition receptors . The receptors for innate immune system are developed at the level of germline (adaptive are generated by somatic recombination). The innate immunity does not react with the normal and healthy cells.

Toll Like Receptors

Toll like receptors (TLRs) are the families of PAMP expressed in many cell types and are involved in the recognition of various kind of antigens. The gene for TLR was first discovered in Drosophila. There are nine different kinds of TLRs (TLR1-9) each recognizing different antigenic molecules. TLR contains leucine repeats and cysteine rich motif at their extracellular domain while intracellular domain contains toll IL-1 receptor (TIR). The extracellular part of TLR is involved in ligand binding while the intracellular domains are involved in the downstream signaling cascade.

Figure: Structure of Toll like receptor:

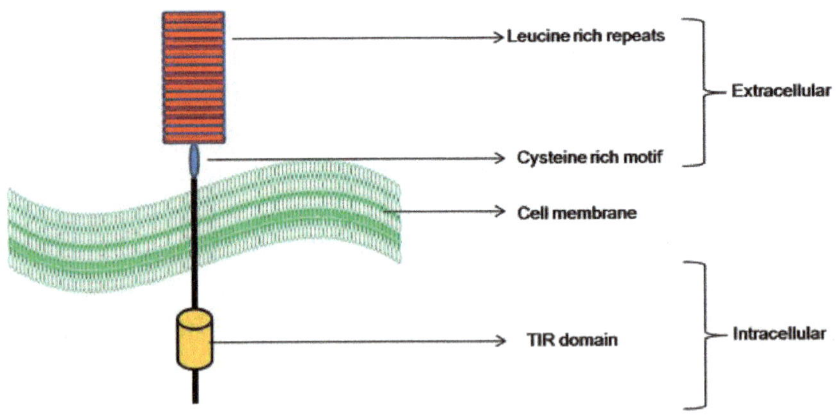

TLRs are found in the cell surface as well as inside the cells and hence are able to recognize a wide variety of antigens. TLR-1, -2, -4, -5 and -6 are expressed over the surface of plasma membrane while TLR-3, -7, -8, and -9 are expressed inside endosomal membrane. Different TLRs can recognize different antigens as listed below.

TLR-1 Bacterial lipoprotein

TLR-2 Bacterial peptidoglycans

TLR-3 Double stranded RNA

TLR-4 Lipopolysaccharides

TLR-5 Bacterial flagella

TLR-6 Bacterial lipoprotein

TLR-7 Single stranded RNA

TLR-8 Single stranded RNA

TLR-9 CpG DNA

Figure: Location of Toll like receptor:

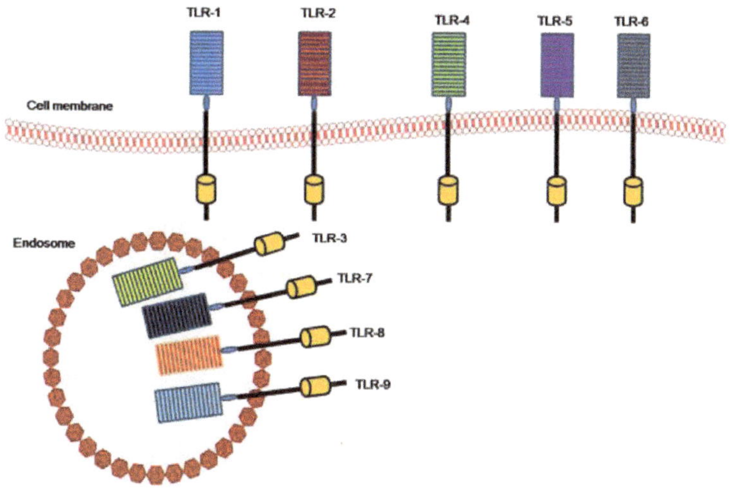

Signaling pathway of TLR activation begins with the ligand binding either on the cell surface or in the endosome. The binding of ligand to TLR leads to dimerization of the TLR which further recruits the adaptor proteins such as MyD88. The adaptor proteins then activate the transcription factor such as NF-κβ, activation protein-1, interferon response factor-3 (IRF-3) and IRF-7. NF-κβ and activation protein-1stimulates the production of inflammatory cytokines (TNF and IL-1) while IRF-3 and -7 promote the production of type-I interferon.

Receptors for PAMPs and DAMPs Present in Cytosol

In addition to membrane bound TLR many receptors are present in the cytosol which can sense the invading antigenic structures.

Nucleotide oligomerization domain (NOD) like receptors present in the cytosol is specialized to sense PAMP and DAMP and recruit the chemical mediators of inflammation. NOD1 can sense invading gram negative bacteria while NOD2 can recognize the muramyl dipeptide from both gram positive and negative bacteria.

Retinoic acid-inducible gene-I (RIG-I) like receptors are another sensors present in the cytosol which are specific against viral RNA and induce the production of type I interferon.

Carbohydrates present on the surface of microbes are recognized by C-type lectin receptors and facilitate their phagocytosis. Similarly, mannose receptors are also playing an important role in sensing the carbohydrate entity present over the surface of many microorganisms. Another group of receptor called dendritic cell-associated C type lectin-1 (Dectin-1) and dectin-2 are important sensors of fungal antigens.

In addition, many cell types express different receptors involved in the phagocytosis of the antigens. Scavenger receptors present over the surface of macrophages senses specifically the oxidized lipoproteins from bacterial cell. N-formyl met-leu-phe receptors are expressed over the surface of neutrophils and macrophages and are involved in the recognition of the N formylmethionyl residues of bacterial origin.

Cellular Components

Many different cellular components are involved in the proper functioning of the body innate immune system.

1. Epithelial cells

   Epithelial cells over the skin surface are the physical barriers for the invading pathogens. Epithelial cells produce antimicrobial substances such as defensins and cathelicidins which also hinder the entry of pathogens. Epithelial barriers include skin, gastrointestinal and respiratory mucosa. Intraepithelial T lymphocytes present in the skin and gastrointestinal tract can respond to the encountering pathogens.

2. Phagocytes

   Macrophages and neutrophils are the first line of defense against the pathogens and are specialized in phagocytic function. Usually phagocytic cells are involved in killing of the microbes and secretion of cytokines that mediate the inflammatory response.

3. Dendritic cells

   They are one of the most important components of the innate immune system. Their role of presenting the antigens to the cells of adaptive immune system makes it unique among the others. They express variety of TLRs, PAMPs and DAMPs for the recognition of the pathogens and present it to the naïve T lymphocytes to trigger the adaptive immune response.

Soluble Components of Innate Immune System

The soluble components of innate immune system bind with the microbes and help in their phagocytosis by the cells of innate immunity. They may sometimes involve in direct killing of the pathogens by promoting the inflammatory response.

Complement System

This system consists of many plasma proteins that help in opsonization of the microbial antigens to promote the recruitment of phagocytic cells. It involves a cascade in which an inactive zymogen is converted into active proteases and many proteolytic products.

First step in the activation of complement system is the recognition of the foreign substance and that occurs by three different pathways

1. Classical pathway
2. Alternate pathway
3. Lectin pathway

Classical pathway was named as it was discovered first and uses the plasma protein C1q to detect antibody bound over the surface of microbes. Following the binding, C1q starts the cascade which leads to lysis of the microbes. Alternate pathway is triggered with a protein called C3 which recognizes the lipopolysaccharides present in the bacterial cell. Lectin pathway is triggered by the mannose binding lectin that recognizes the mannose residues present in the microbes.

Recognition of antigens by any of these pathways converts C3 into C3a and C3b with the help of C3 convertase. C3b binds with the microbial antigen while C3a stimulates the release of inflammatory cytokines. C3b activates the C5 convertase to convert C5 into C5a and C5b. C5a is a chemoattractant while C5b initiates the formation of complex with other complement proteins C6, C7, C8, and C9. This sequential cascade leads to formation of membrane attack complex which causes lysis of the cell.

Figure: Complement system pathways:

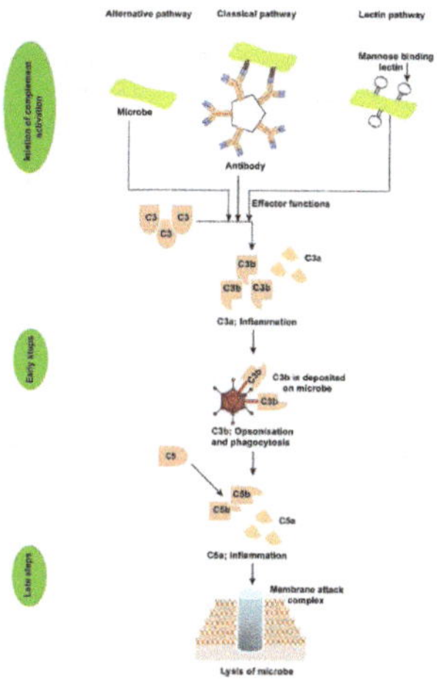

References

- Janeway, C.A.; Travers, P.; Walport, M.; Shlomchik, M.J. (2005). Immunobiology. (6th ed.). Garland Science. ISBN 0-443-07310-4
- "Study of VX-765 in Subjects With Treatment-resistant Partial Epilepsy - Full Text View - ClinicalTrials.gov". clinicaltrials.gov. Retrieved 2016-05-21
- Abbas A.B.; Lichtman A.H. (2009). "Ch.2 Innate Immunity". In Saunders (Elsevier). Basic Immunology. Functions and disorders of the immune system (3rd ed.). ISBN 978-1-4160-4688-2
- M Stitzinger (2007). "Lipids, inflammation and atherosclerosis" (pdf). The digital repository of Leiden University. Retrieved 2007-11-02
- Eming, S. A.; Krieg, T.; Davidson, J. M. (2007). "Inflammation in wound repair: molecular and cellular mechanisms". Journal of Investigative Dermatology. 127 (3): 514–525. doi:10.1038/sj.jid.5700701. PMID 17299434
- Hall, John (2011). Guyton and Hall textbook of medical physiology (12th ed.). Philadelphia, Pa.: Saunders/Elsevier. p. 428. ISBN 978-1-4160-4574-8
- Shih, Michael. "Skeletal Muscle Hypertrophy Is Regulated via AKT/mTOR Pathway." BioCarta. Web. 21 March 2011. "Archived copy". Archived from the original on 14 September 2010. Retrieved 2011-03-21
- Cotran; Kumar, Collins (1998). Robbins Pathologic Basis of Disease. Philadelphia: W.B Saunders Company. ISBN 0-7216-7335-X
- Vogel, Wolfgang H.; Berke, Andreas (2009). Brief History of Vision and Ocular Medicine. Kugler Publications. p. 97. ISBN 90-6299-220-X
- "Appendicitis". National Institute of Diabetes and Digestive and Kidney Diseases. U.S Department of Health and Human Services. Retrieved 2010-02-01
- Hawke, TJ; Garry, DJ (Aug 2001). "Myogenic satellite cells: physiology to molecular biology.". Journal of applied physiology (Bethesda, Md. : 1985). 91 (2): 534–51. PMID 11457764
- Porth, Carol (2007). Essentials of pahtophysiology: concepts of altered health states. Hagerstown, MD: Lippincott Williams & Wilkins. p. 270. ISBN 0-7817-7087-4
- "WHO Disease and injury country estimates". World Health Organization. 2009. Archived from the original on 11 November 2009. Retrieved Nov 11, 2009
- Jurasinski, CV; Vary, TC (Nov 1995). "Insulin-like growth factor I accelerates protein synthesis in skeletal muscle during sepsis.". The American journal of physiology. 269 (5 Pt 1): E977–81. PMID 7491951
- Dormandy, Thomas (2006). The worst of evils: man's fight against pain. New Haven, Conn: Yale University Press. p. 22. ISBN 0-300-11322-6
- Vary, TC; Kimball, SR (Feb 1992). "Regulation of hepatic protein synthesis in chronic inflammation and sepsis.". The American journal of physiology. 262 (2 Pt 1): C445–52. PMID 1371643
- Pedersen, BK (Jul 2013). "Muscle as a secretory organ". Comprehensive Physiology. 3 (3): 1337–62. doi:10.1002/cphy.c120033. ISBN 9780470650714. PMID 23897689

3

An Overview of Adaptive Immune System

While the innate system is the more primitive defense against infections, the adaptive immune system provides long-lasting immunity. This system creates a memory of response to an attack, which helps in providing an improved response to similar future attacks. The two major constituents of adaptive immune system are antibodies and antigens. The topics discussed in the chapter are of great importance to broaden the existing knowledge on adaptive immune system.

Adaptive Immune System

The adaptive immune system, also known as the acquired immune system or, more rarely, as the specific immune system, is a subsystem of the overall immune system that is composed of highly specialized, systemic cells and processes that eliminate pathogens or prevent their growth. The adaptive immune system is one of the two main immunity strategies found in vertebrates (the other being the innate immune system). Adaptive immunity creates immunological memory after an initial response to a specific pathogen, and leads to an enhanced response to subsequent encounters with that pathogen. This process of acquired immunity is the basis of vaccination. Like the innate system, the adaptive system includes both humoral immunity components and cell-mediated immunity components.

Unlike the innate immune system, the adaptive immune system is highly specific to a particular pathogen. Adaptive immunity can also provide long-lasting protection; for example, someone who recovers from measles is now protected against measles for their lifetime. In other cases it does not provide lifetime protection; for example, chickenpox. The adaptive system response destroys invading pathogens and any toxic molecules they produce. Sometimes the adaptive system is unable to distinguish harmful from harmless foreign molecules; the effects of this may be hayfever, asthma or any other allergy. Antigens are any substances that elicit the adaptive immune response. The cells that carry out the adaptive immune response are white blood cells known as lymphocytes. Two main broad classes—antibody responses and cell mediated immune response—are also carried by two different lymphocytes (B cells and T cells). In antibody responses, B cells are activated to secrete antibodies, which are proteins also known as immunoglobulins. Antibodies travel through the bloodstream and bind to the foreign antigen causing it to inactivate, which does not allow the antigen to bind to the host.

In acquired immunity, pathogen-specific receptors are "acquired" during the lifetime of the organism (whereas in innate immunity pathogen-specific receptors are already encoded in the germline). The acquired response is called "adaptive" because it prepares the body's immune system for future challenges (though it can actually also be maladaptive when it results in autoimmunity).

The system is highly adaptable because of somatic hypermutation (a process of accelerated somatic mutations), and V(D)J recombination (an irreversible genetic recombination of antigen receptor gene segments). This mechanism allows a small number of genes to generate a vast number of different antigen receptors, which are then uniquely expressed on each individual lymphocyte. Since the gene rearrangement leads to an irreversible change in the DNA of each cell, all progeny (offspring) of that cell inherit genes that encode the same receptor specificity, including the memory B cells and memory T cells that are the keys to long-lived specific immunity.

A theoretical framework explaining the workings of the adaptive immune system is provided by immune network theory. This theory, which builds on established concepts of clonal selection, is being applied in the search for an HIV vaccine.

Functions

Adaptive immunity is triggered in vertebrates when a pathogen evades the innate immune system and (1) generates a threshold level of antigen and (2) generates "stranger" or "danger" signals activating dendritic cells.

The major functions of the adaptive immune system include:

- Recognition of specific "non-self" antigens in the presence of "self", during the process of antigen presentation.
- Generation of responses that are tailored to maximally eliminate specific pathogens or pathogen-infected cells.
- Development of immunological memory, in which pathogens are "remembered" through memory B cells and memory T cells.

Lymphocytes

The cells of the adaptive immune system are T and B lymphocytes; lymphocytes are a subset of leukocyte. B cells and T cells are the major types of lymphocytes. The human body has about 2 trillion lymphocytes, constituting 20–40% of white blood cells (WBCs); their total mass is about the same as the brain or liver. The peripheral blood contains 2% of circulating lymphocytes; the rest move within the tissues and lymphatic system.

B cells and T cells are derived from the same multipotent hematopoietic stem cells, and are morphologically indistinguishable from one another until after they are activated. B cells play a large role in the humoral immune response, whereas T cells are intimately involved in cell-mediated immune responses. In all vertebrates except Agnatha, B cells and T cells are produced by stem cells in the bone marrow.

T progenitors migrate from the bone marrow to the thymus where they are called thymocytes and where they develop into T cells. In humans, approximately 1–2% of the lymphocyte pool recirculates each hour to optimize the opportunities for antigen-specific lymphocytes to find their specific antigen within the secondary lymphoid tissues. In an adult animal, the peripheral lymphoid organs contain a mixture of B and T cells in at least three stages of differentiation:

- naive B and naive T cells (cells that have not matured), left the bone marrow or thymus, have entered the lymphatic system, but have yet to encounter their cognate antigen,
- effector cells that have been activated by their cognate antigen, and are actively involved in eliminating a pathogen.
- memory cells – the survivors of past infections.

Antigen Presentation

Adaptive immunity relies on the capacity of immune cells to distinguish between the body's own cells and unwanted invaders. The host's cells express "self" antigens. These antigens are different from those on the surface of bacteria or on the surface of virus-infected host cells ("non-self" or "foreign" antigens). The adaptive immune response is triggered by recognizing foreign antigen in the cellular context of an activated dendritic cell.

With the exception of non-nucleated cells (including erythrocytes), all cells are capable of presenting antigen through the function of major histocompatibility complex (MHC) molecules. Some cells are specially equipped to present antigen, and to prime naive T cells. Dendritic cells, B-cells, and macrophages are equipped with special "co-stimulatory" ligands recognized by co-stimulatory receptors on T cells, and are termed professional antigen-presenting cells (APCs).

Several T cells subgroups can be activated by professional APCs, and each type of T cell is specially equipped to deal with each unique toxin or microbial pathogen. The type of T cell activated, and the type of response generated, depends, in part, on the context in which the APC first encountered the antigen.

Exogenous Antigens

Dendritic cells engulf exogenous pathogens, such as bacteria, parasites or toxins in the tissues and then migrate, via chemotactic signals, to the T cell-enriched lymph nodes. During migration, dendritic cells undergo a process of maturation in which they lose most of their ability to engulf other pathogens and develop an ability to communicate with T-cells. The dendritic cell uses enzymes to chop the pathogen into smaller pieces, called antigens. In the lymph node, the dendritic cell displays these non-self antigens on its surface by coupling them to a receptor called the major histocompatibility complex, or MHC (also known in humans as human leukocyte antigen (HLA)). This MHC:antigen complex is recognized by T-cells passing through the lymph node. Exogenous antigens are usually displayed on MHC class II molecules, which activate CD4+T helper cells.

Endogenous Antigens

Endogenous antigens are produced by intracellular bacteria and viruses replicating within a host cell.The host cell uses enzymes to digest virally associated proteins, and displays these pieces on its surface to T-cells by coupling them to MHC. Endogenous antigens are typically displayed on MHC class I molecules, and activate CD8+ cytotoxic T-cells. With the exception of non-nucleated cells (including erythrocytes), MHC class I is expressed by all host cells.

CD8+ T Lymphocytes and Cytotoxicity

Cytotoxic T cells (also known as TC, killer T cell, or cytotoxic T-lymphocyte (CTL)) are a sub-group of T cells that induce the death of cells that are infected with viruses (and other pathogens), or are otherwise damaged or dysfunctional.

Naive cytotoxic T cells are activated when their T-cell receptor (TCR) strongly interacts with a peptide-bound MHC class I molecule. This affinity depends on the type and orientation of the antigen/MHC complex, and is what keeps the CTL and infected cell bound together. Once activated, the CTL undergoes a process called clonal selection, in which it gains functions and divides rapidly to produce an army of "armed" effector cells. Activated CTL then travels throughout the body searching for cells that bear that unique MHC Class I + peptide.

When exposed to these infected or dysfunctional somatic cells, effector CTL release perforin and granulysin: cytotoxins that form pores in the target cell's plasma membrane, allowing ions and water to flow into the infected cell, and causing it to burst or lyse. CTL release granzyme, a serine protease that enters cells via pores to induce apoptosis (cell death). To limit extensive tissue damage during an infection, CTL activation is tightly controlled and in general requires a very strong MHC/antigen activation signal, or additional activation signals provided by "helper" T-cells.

On resolution of the infection, most effector cells die and phagocytes clear them away—but a few of these cells remain as memory cells. On a later encounter with the same antigen, these memory cells quickly differentiate into effector cells, dramatically shortening the time required to mount an effective response.

Helper T-cells

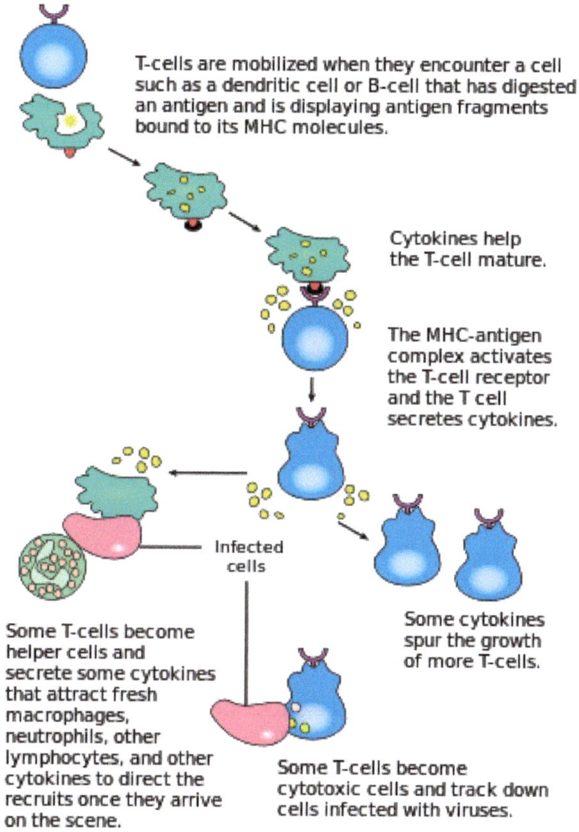

The T lymphocyte activation pathway. T cells contribute to immune defenses in two major ways: some direct and regulate immune responses; others directly attack infected or cancerous cells.

CD4+ lymphocytes, also called "helper" or "regulatory" T cells, are immune response mediators, and play an important role in establishing and maximizing the capabilities of the adaptive immune response. These cells have no cytotoxic or phagocytic activity; and cannot kill infected cells or clear pathogens, but, in essence "manage" the immune response, by directing other cells to perform these tasks.

Helper T cells express T cell receptors (TCR) that recognize antigen bound to Class II MHC molecules. The activation of a naive helper T-cell causes it to release cytokines, which influences the activity of many cell types, including the APC (Antigen-Presenting Cell) that activated it. Helper T-cells require a much milder activation stimulus than cytotoxic T cells. Helper T cells can provide extra signals that "help" activate cytotoxic cells.

Th1 and Th2: Helper T Cell Responses

Classically, two types of effector CD4+ T helper cell responses can be induced by a professional APC, designated Th1 and Th2, each designed to eliminate different types of pathogens. The factors that dictate whether an infection triggers a Th1 or Th2 type response are not fully understood, but the response generated does play an important role in the clearance of different pathogens.

The Th1 response is characterized by the production of Interferon-gamma, which activates the bactericidal activities of macrophages, and induces B cells to make opsonizing (coating) and complement-fixing antibodies, and leads to *cell-mediated immunity*. In general, Th1 responses are more effective against intracellular pathogens (viruses and bacteria that are inside host cells).

The Th2 response is characterized by the release of Interleukin 5, which induces eosinophils in the clearance of parasites. Th2 also produce Interleukin 4, which facilitates B cell isotype switching. In general, Th2 responses are more effective against extracellular bacteria, parasites including helminths and toxins. Like cytotoxic T cells, most of the CD4+ helper cells die on resolution of infection, with a few remaining as CD4+ memory cells.

Increasingly, there is strong evidence from mouse and human-based scientific studies of a broader diversity in CD4+ effector T helper cell subsets. Regulatory T (Treg) cells, have been identified as important negative regulators of adaptive immunity as they limit and suppresses the immune system to control aberrant immune responses to self-antigens; an important mechanism in controlling the development of autoimmune diseases. Follicular helper T (Tfh) cells are another distinct population of effector CD4+ T cells that develop from naive T cells post-antigen activation. Tfh cells are specialized in helping B cell humoral immunity as they are uniquely capable of migrating to follicular B cells in secondary lymphoid organs and provide them positive paracrine signals to enable the generation and recall production of high-quality affinity-matured antibodies. Similar to Tregs, Tfh cells also play a role in immunological tolerance as an abnormal expansion of Tfh cell numbers can lead to unrestricted autoreactive antibody production causing severe systemic autoimmune disorders.

The relevance of CD4+ T helper cells is highlighted during an HIV infection. HIV is able to subvert the immune system by specifically attacking the CD4+ T cells, precisely the cells that could drive the clearance of the virus, but also the cells that drive immunity against all other pathogens encountered during an organism's lifetime.

Gamma Delta T Cells

Gamma delta T cells (γδ T cells) possess an alternative T cell receptor (TCR) as opposed to CD4+ and CD8+ αβ T cells and share characteristics of helper T cells, cytotoxic T cells and natural killer cells. Like other 'unconventional' T cell subsets bearing invariant TCRs, such as CD1d-restricted natural killer T cells, γδ T cells exhibit characteristics that place them at the border between innate and adaptive immunity. On one hand, γδ T cells may be considered a component of adaptive immunity in that they rearrange TCR genes via V(D)J recombination, which also produces junctional diversity, and develop a memory phenotype. On the other hand, however, the various subsets may also be considered part of the innate immune system where a restricted TCR or NK receptors may be used as a pattern recognition receptor. For example, according to this paradigm, large numbers of Vγ9/Vδ2 T cells respond within hours to common molecules produced by microbes, and highly restricted intraepithelial Vδ1 T cells respond to stressed epithelial cells.

B Lymphocytes and Antibody Production

B Cells are the major cells involved in the creation of antibodies that circulate in blood plasma and lymph, known as humoral immunity. Antibodies (also known as immunoglobulin, Ig), are large Y-shaped proteins used by the immune system to identify and neutralize foreign objects. In mammals, there are five types of antibody: IgA, IgD, IgE, IgG, and IgM, differing in biological properties; each has evolved to handle different kinds of antigens. Upon activation, B cells produce antibodies, each of which recognizing a unique antigen, and neutralizing specific pathogens.

Like the T cell, B cells express a unique B cell receptor (BCR), in this case, a membrane-bound antibody molecule. All the BCR of any one clone of B cells recognizes and binds to only one particular antigen. A critical difference between B cells and T cells is how each cell “sees” an antigen. T cells recognize their cognate antigen in a processed form – as a peptide in the context of an MHC molecule, whereas B cells recognize antigens in their native form. Once a B cell encounters its cognate (or specific) antigen (and receives additional signals from a helper T cell (predominately Th2 type)), it further differentiates into an effector cell, known as a plasma cell.

Plasma cells are short-lived cells (2–3 days) that secrete antibodies. These antibodies bind to antigens, making them easier targets for phagocytes, and trigger the complement cascade. About 10% of plasma cells survive to become long-lived antigen-specific memory B cells. Already primed to produce specific antibodies, these cells can be called upon to respond quickly if the same pathogen re-infects the host, while the host experiences few, if any, symptoms.

Alternative Adaptive Immune System

Although the classical molecules of the adaptive immune system (e.g., antibodies and T cell receptors) exist only in jawed vertebrates, a distinct lymphocyte-derived molecule has been discovered in primitive jawless vertebrates, such as the lamprey and hagfish. These animals possess a large array of molecules called variable lymphocyte receptors (VLRs for short) that, like the antigen receptors of jawed vertebrates, are produced from only a small number (one or two) of genes. These molecules are believed to bind pathogenic antigens in a similar way to antibodies, and with the same degree of specificity.

Immunological Memory

When B cells and T cells are activated some become memory B cells and some memory T cells. Throughout the lifetime of an animal these memory cells form a database of effective B and T lymphocytes. Upon interaction with a previously encountered antigen, the appropriate memory cells are selected and activated. In this manner, the second and subsequent exposures to an antigen produce a stronger and faster immune response. This is "adaptive" because the body's immune system prepares itself for future challenges, but is "maladaptive" of course if the receptors are autoimmune. Immunological memory can be in the form of either *passive* short-term memory or *active* long-term memory.

Passive Memory

Passive memory is usually short-term, lasting between a few days and several months. Newborn infants have had no prior exposure to microbes and are particularly vulnerable to infection. Several layers of passive protection are provided by the mother. *In utero*, maternal IgG is transported directly across the placenta, so that, at birth, human babies have high levels of antibodies, with the same range of antigen specificities as their mother. Breast milk contains antibodies (mainly IgA) that are transferred to the gut of the infant, protecting against bacterial infections, until the newborn can synthesize its own antibodies.

This is passive immunity because the fetus does not actually make any memory cells or antibodies: It only borrows them. Short-term passive immunity can also be transferred artificially from one individual to another via antibody-rich serum.

Active Memory

In general, active immunity is long-term and can be acquired by infection followed by B cells and T cells activation, or artificially acquired by vaccines, in a process called immunization.

Immunization

Historically, infectious disease has been the leading cause of death in the human population. Over the last century, two important factors have been developed to combat their spread: sanitation and immunization. Immunization (commonly referred to as vaccination) is the deliberate induction of an immune response, and represents the single most effective manipulation of the immune system that scientists have developed. Immunizations are successful because they utilize the immune system's natural specificity as well as its inducibility.

The principle behind immunization is to introduce an antigen, derived from a disease-causing organism, that stimulates the immune system to develop protective immunity against that organism, but that does not itself cause the pathogenic effects of that organism. An antigen (short for *anti*body *gen*erator), is defined as any substance that binds to a specific antibody and elicits an adaptive immune response.

Most viral vaccines are based on live attenuated viruses, whereas many bacterial vaccines are based on acellular components of microorganisms, including harmless toxin components. Many antigens derived from acellular vaccines do not strongly induce an adaptive response, and most bacterial vaccines require the addition of *adjuvants* that activate the antigen-presenting cells of the innate immune system to enhance immunogenicity.

Immunological Diversity

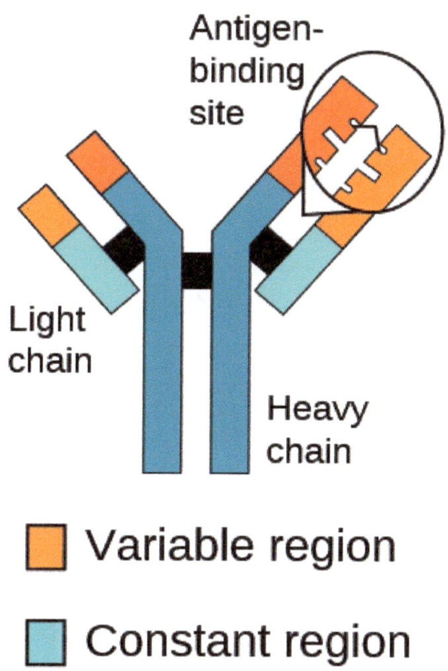

An antibody is made up of two heavy chains and two light chains. The unique variable region allows an antibody to recognize its matching antigen.

Most large molecules, including virtually all proteins and many polysaccharides, can serve as antigens. The parts of an antigen that interact with an antibody molecule or a lymphocyte receptor, are called epitopes, or antigenic determinants. Most antigens contain a variety of epitopes and can stimulate the production of antibodies, specific T cell responses, or both. A very small proportion (less than 0.01%) of the total lymphocytes are able to bind to a particular antigen, which suggests that only a few cells respond to each antigen.

For the adaptive response to "remember" and eliminate a large number of pathogens the immune system must be able to distinguish between many different antigens, and the receptors that recognize antigens must be produced in a huge variety of configurations, in essence one receptor (at least) for each different pathogen that might ever be encountered. Even in the absence of antigen stimulation, a human can produce more than 1 trillion different antibody molecules. Millions of genes would be required to store the genetic information that produces these receptors, but, the entire human genome contains fewer than 25,000 genes.

Myriad receptors are produced through a process known as clonal selection. According to the clonal selection theory, at birth, an animal randomly generates a vast diversity of lymphocytes (each bearing a unique antigen receptor) from information encoded in a small family of genes. To generate each unique antigen receptor, these genes have undergone a process called V(D)J recombination, or *combinatorial diversification*, in which one gene segment recombines with other gene segments to form a single unique gene. This assembly process generates the enormous diversity of receptors and antibodies, before the body ever encounters antigens, and enables the immune system to respond to an almost unlimited diversity of antigens. Throughout an animal's lifetime, lymphocytes that can react against the antigens an animal actually encounters are selected for action—directed against anything that expresses that antigen.

Note that the innate and adaptive portions of the immune system work together, not in spite of each other. The adaptive arm, B, and T cells couldn't function without the innate system' input. T cells are useless without antigen-presenting cells to activate them, and B cells are crippled without T cell help. On the other hand, the innate system would likely be overrun with pathogens without the specialized action of the adaptive immune response.

Adaptive Immunity During Pregnancy

The cornerstone of the immune system is the recognition of "self" versus "non-self". Therefore, the mechanisms that protect the human fetus (which is considered "non-self") from attack by the immune system, are particularly interesting. Although no comprehensive explanation has emerged to explain this mysterious, and often repeated, lack of rejection, two classical reasons may explain how the fetus is tolerated. The first is that the fetus occupies a portion of the body protected by a non-immunological barrier, the uterus, which the immune system does not routinely patrol. The second is that the fetus itself may promote local immunosuppression in the mother, perhaps by a process of active nutrient depletion. A more modern explanation for this induction of tolerance is that specific glycoproteins expressed in the uterus during pregnancy suppress the uterine immune response.

During pregnancy in viviparous mammals (all mammals except Monotremes), endogenous retroviruses (ERVs) are activated and produced in high quantities during the implantation of the embryo. They are currently known to possess immunosuppressive properties, suggesting a role in protecting the embryo from its mother's immune system. Also, viral fusion proteins cause the formation of the placental syncytium to limit exchange of migratory cells between the developing embryo and the body of the mother (something an epithelium can't do sufficiently, as certain blood cells specialize to insert themselves between adjacent epithelial cells). The immunodepressive action was the initial normal behavior of the virus, similar to HIV. The fusion proteins were a way to spread the infection to other cells by simply merging them with the infected one (HIV does this too). It is believed that the ancestors of modern viviparous mammals evolved after an infection by this virus, enabling the fetus to survive the immune system of the mother.

The human genome project found several thousand ERVs classified into 24 families.

Immune Network Theory

A theoretical framework explaining the workings of the adaptive immune system is provided by immune network theory, based on interactions between idiotypes (unique molecular features of one clonotype, i.e. the unique set of antigenic determinants of the variable portion of an antibody) and 'anti-idiotypes' (antigen receptors that react with the idiotype as if it were a foreign antigen). This theory, which builds on the existing clonal selection hypothesis and since 1974 has been developed mainly by Niels Jerne and Geoffrey W. Hoffmann, is seen as being relevant to the understanding of the HIV pathogenesis and the search for an HIV vaccine.

Stimulation of Adaptive Immunity

One of the most interesting developments in biomedical science during the past few decades has been elucidation of mechanisms mediating innate immunity. One set of innate immune mechanisms is humoral, such as complement activation. Another set comprises pattern recognition receptors such as toll-like receptors, which induce the production of interferons and other cytokines increasing resistance of cells such as monocytes to infections. Cytokines produced during innate immune responses are among the activators of adaptive immune responses. Antibodies exert additive or synergistic effects with mechanisms of innate immunity. Unstable HbS clusters Band-3, a major integral red cell protein; antibodies recognize these clusters and accelerate their removal by phagocytic cells. Clustered Band 3 proteins with attached antibodies activate complement, and complement C3 fragments are opsonins recognized by the CR1 complement receptor on phagocytic cells.

A population study has shown that the protective effect of the sickle-cell trait against falciparum malaria involves the augmentation of adaptive as well as innate immune responses to the malaria parasite, illustrating the expected transition from innate to adaptive immunity.

Repeated malaria infections strengthen adaptive immunity and broaden its effects against parasites expressing different surface antigens. By school age most children have developed efficacious adaptive immunity against malaria. These observations raise questions about mechanisms that favor the survival of most children in Africa while allowing some to develop potentially lethal infections.

In malaria, as in other infections, innate immune responses lead into, and stimulate, adaptive immune responses. The genetic control of innate and adaptive immunity is now a large and flourishing discipline.

Humoral and cell-mediated immune responses limit malaria parasite multiplication, and many cytokines contribute to the pathogenesis of malaria as well as to the resolution of infections.

Evolution

The adaptive immune system, which has been best-studied in mammals, originated in jawed fish approximately 500 million years ago. Most of the molecules, cells, tissues, and associated mechanisms of this system of defense are found in cartilaginous fishes. Lymphocyte receptors, Ig and TCR, are found in all jawed vertebrates. The most ancient Ig class, IgM, is membrane-bound and then secreted upon stimulation of cartilaginous fish B cells. Another isotype, shark IgW, is related to mammalian IgD. TCRs, both α/β and γ/δ, are found in all animals from gnathostomes to mammals. The organization of gene segments that undergo gene rearrangement differs in cartilaginous fishes, which have a cluster form as compared to the translocon form in bony fish to mammals. Like TCR and Ig, the MHC is found only in jawed vertebrates. Genes involved in antigen processing and presentation, as well as the class I and class II genes, are closely linked within the MHC of almost all studied species.

Lymphoid cells can be identified in some pre-vertebrate deuterostomes (i.e., sea urchins). These bind antigen with pattern recognition receptors (PRRs) of the innate immune system. In jawless fishes, two subsets of lymphocytes use variable lymphocyte receptors (VLRs) for antigen binding. Diversity is generated by a cytosine deaminase-mediated rearrangement of LRR-based DNA segments. There is no evidence for the recombination-activating genes (RAGs) that rearrange Ig and TCR gene segments in jawed vertebrates.

The evolution of the AIS, based on Ig, TCR, and MHC molecules, is thought to have arisen from two major evolutionary events: the transfer of the RAG transposon (possibly of viral origin) and two whole genome duplications. Though the molecules of the AIS are well-conserved, they are also rapidly evolving. Yet, a comparative approach finds that many features are quite uniform across taxa. All the major features of the AIS arose early and quickly. Jawless fishes have a different AIS that relies on gene rearrangement to generate diversity but has little else in common with the jawed vertebrate AIS. The innate immune system, which has an important role in AIS activation, is the most important defense system of invertebrates and plants.

Cell Mediated Immune Response

This is also called cellular immunity, and is mediated by T lymphocytes. Cell mediated immunity plays an important role against intracellular microbes, viruses, and some intracellular bacteria. The cellular immunity promotes the destruction of microbes by direct killing or phagocytosis of the infected cells.

Figure: Schematic representation of humoral and cell mediated immunity:

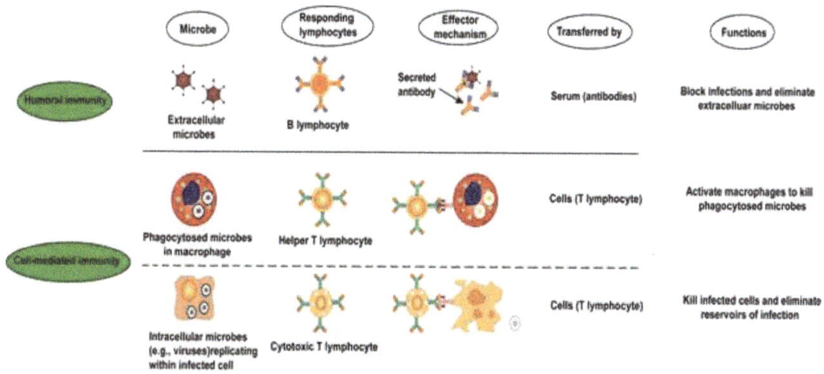

Immunity against a pathogen is usually induced by the exposure of microbial antigen to the host and is called active immunity. Immunity can also be transferred by serum or lymphocyte from an immunized individual to a diseased individual and is called passive immunity . Passive immunization is a rapid way to transfer the immunity in the absence of active immunity. Passive immunization against toxin and venoms is a life saving treatment in many lethal conditions (Tetanus toxoid, snake antivenom).

Figure: Schematic representation of active and passive immunity:

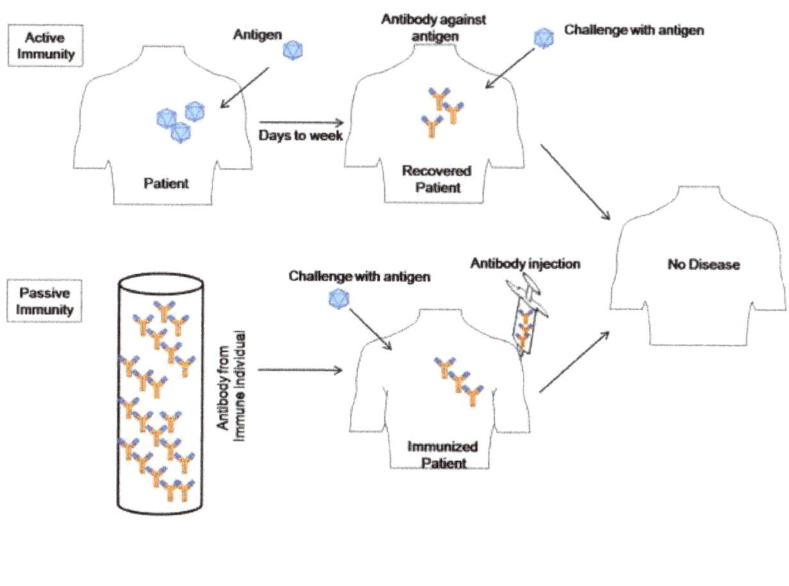

The first concept of humoral immunity was given by Emil von Behring and Shibasabro Kitasato ; they showed for the first time that serum transferred from a recovered diphtheria patient protected the recipient from active diphtheria infection. The active ingredients are called antitoxins because they nullify the effect of toxins. They won the noble prize for their landmark discovery. Paul Ehrlich coined the term antibodies for the proteins present in the serum and showed that it is capable to bind and neutralize the toxins. The substances that induce the production of antibodies are called antigens . The definition of the antigen changed in due course of time with the modern discoveries. The antigens are defined as substances that bind to a specific lymphocyte with or without further production of antibody. However the substances that induce the production of antibodies are called immunogens in modern immunology world.

The cellular theory of immunity started with the work of Elie Metchnikoff , who first demonstrated the phenomenon of phagocytosis. Another remarkable finding was put forth by Almroth Wright, who showed that the factors present in the serum can coat the bacteria and help them to phagocytize by the cells of the immune system, the process known as opsonization.

Feature of Adaptive Immunity

The adaptive immunity has some fundamental properties.

1. Specificity : The adaptive immunity is specific to a particular antigen, which means specific antibodies are produced against a particular antigen. The structures present over the antigen that stimulate the production of antibodies are called antigenic determinants or epitopes . Minute differences exist among lymphocytes that express membrane receptors which are able to distinguish fine differences present on the epitopes. The specificity of immune system leads to a huge population of lymphocytes that are antigenically specific and are called lymphocyte repertoire.

2. Diversity : The ability of lymphocyte repertoire to recognize a wide variety of antigens is called diversity. In fact lymphocyte repertoire that contains receptors for different antigen contributes to a large population of extremely diverse lymphocyte clones.

3. Memory : The ability of the immune system to remember the antigens and respond again to the same upon exposure is called immunological memory. The immune response against the second exposure of the same antigen or subsequent exposure is usually rapid and larger than the primary immune response.

Figure: Memory response of the adaptive immune system:

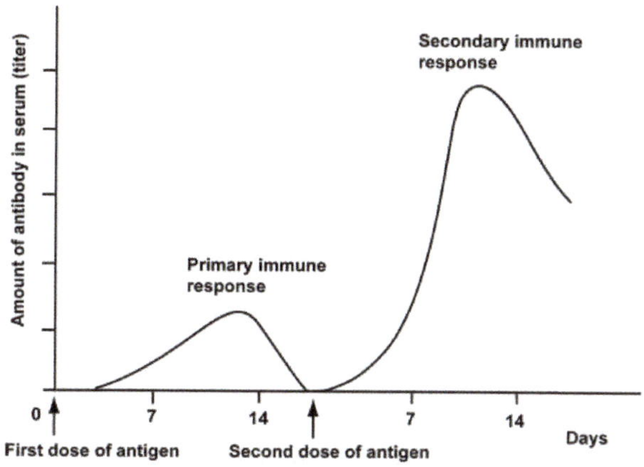

Immunologic memory forms because of long-lived memory cells generated upon each exposure of an antigen and are specific for that antigen. The memory cells produced following second exposure are more efficient in eliminating the antigen as compared to the primary immune response.

Nonreactivity to Self Antigens

A unique and remarkable property of immune system is to respond and eliminate any foreign antigen (Non self), while not producing any harmful effect against the own antigen (self). It is sometimes called as tolerance towards the self antigen. Any deviation from the above in which immune system starts reacting towards the self antigen leads to a condition what we call as autoimmune diseases.

Specialization

Both humoral and cellular immune system responds to the foreign pathogens in a different way. The responses are different against extracellular and intracellular pathogens. Each type of response is unique for a particular type of pathogen and is specialized to perform specific functions.

Clonal Expansion

It is another unique property of immune system in which the lymphocyte starts producing similar kind of cells upon exposure to an antigen in order to eliminate the pathogen more effectively and more rapidly. The cells formed after clonal expansion has similar surface markers and responds to similar kind of antigen.

Homeostasis

Every process in the body has a regulatory mechanism. The immune responses are produced against an antigen or pathogen upon entry inside the body and wane following the clearance of antigen. This is done in order to maintain homeostasis mechanism inside the body. Any deviation from the homeostasis leads to an immunological disease condition.

Cells of the Adaptive Immune System

Major cells of the adaptive immune system includes following:

- Lymphocytes
- Antigen presenting cells
- Effector cells

Lymphocytes are the main cells which can recognizes the antigen and produce an antibody in order to eliminate the antigens. They are considered as a mediator of both humoral and cellular immunity. B lymphocytes are the only cells in the body capable of producing antibodies. B lymphocytes recognize the extracellular antigens and are differentiated into the plasma cells. T lymphocytes recognize the intracellular antigens and they either help in their phagocytosis or direct killing of the infected cells. T lymphocytes are activated by the antigen loaded over the major histocompatibility complex (MHC) molecules, which are expressed on the surfaces of other cells. T lymphocytes are divided into different subsets which are specific for certain specialized functions. Helper T cells are the subsets of T lymphocyte that secretes the cytokines and help in the proliferation and activation of T lymphocyte. Helper T cells also activate the B cells (to secret the antibody), macrophages and other leucocytes by the virtue of the cytokines. Cytotoxic T lymphocytes kill the cells infected by viruses or other intracellular pathogens. Regulatory T cells help to reduce or inhibit the immune response and are negative regulators of immune system. Natural killer cells are involved in the innate immunity against viruses or other intracellular pathogens. Different classes of lymphocytes can be identified and differentiated by the expression of their surface receptors called cluster of differentiation (CD).

Antigen-presenting cells are mostly the dendritic cells which capture the antigens, transport it to the lymphoid organs and present the antigens to naïve lymphocytes in order to activate the immune response.

Effector cells of the immune system mainly include activated T lymphocytes, mononuclear phagocytes, and other leukocytes. Effector cells are required to complete the immune cascade, i.e. to eliminate the microbes.

Lymphocyte

A lymphocyte is one of the subtypes of white blood cell in a vertebrate's immune system. Lymphocytes include natural killer cells (NK cells) (which function in cell-mediated, cytotoxic innate immunity), T cells (for cell-mediated, cytotoxic adaptive immunity), and B cells (for humoral, antibody-driven adaptive immunity). They are the main type of cell found in lymph, which prompted the name "lymphocyte".

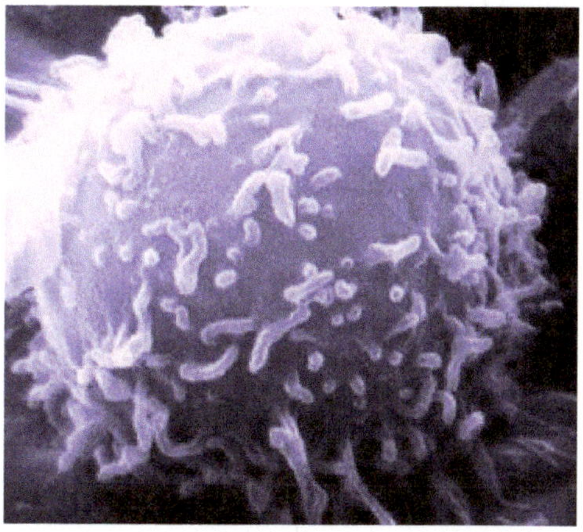

A scanning electron microscope (SEM) image of a single human lymphocyte.

Types

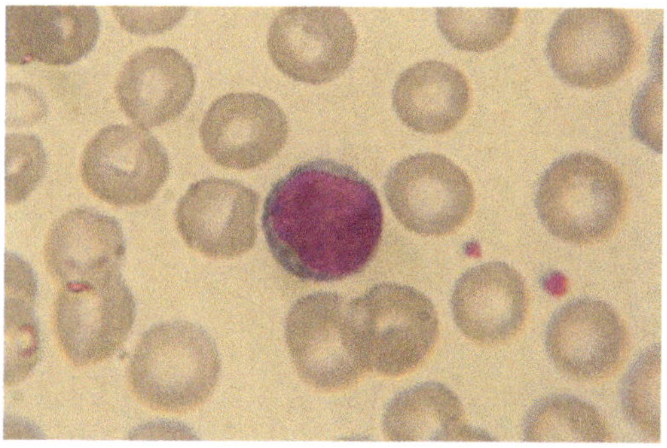

A stained lymphocyte surrounded by red blood cells viewed using a light microscope.

The three major types of lymphocyte are T cells, B cells and natural killer (NK) cells. Lymphocytes can be identified by their large nucleus.

T Cells and B Cells

T cells (thymus cells) and B cells (bone marrow- or bursa-derived cells[a]) are the major cellular components of the adaptive immune response. T cells are involved in cell-mediated immunity, whereas B cells are primarily responsible for humoral immunity (relating to antibodies). The function of T cells and B cells is to recognize specific "non-self" antigens, during a process known as antigen presentation. Once they have identified an invader, the cells generate specific responses that are tailored to maximally eliminate specific pathogens or pathogen-infected cells. B cells respond to pathogens by producing large quantities of antibodies which then neutralize foreign objects like bacteria and viruses. In response to pathogens some T cells, called *T helper cells*, produce cytokines that direct the immune response, while other T cells, called *cytotoxic T cells*, produce toxic granules that contain powerful enzymes which induce the death of pathogen-infected cells. Following activation, B cells and T cells leave a lasting legacy of the antigens they have encountered, in the form of *memory cells*. Throughout the lifetime of an animal, these memory cells will remember each specific pathogen encountered, and are able to mount a strong and rapid response if the same pathogen is detected again; this is known as acquired immunity.

Natural Killer Cells

NK cells are a part of the innate immune system and play a major role in defending the host from both tumors and virally infected cells. NK cells distinguish infected cells and tumors from normal and uninfected cells by recognizing changes of a surface molecule called MHC (major histocompatibility complex) class I. NK cells are activated in response to a family of cytokines called interferons. Activated NK cells release cytotoxic (cell-killing) granules which then destroy the altered cells. They were named "natural killer cells" because of the notion that they do not require prior activation in order to kill cells which are missing MHC class I. This notion seemed doubtful at the time but turned out to be correct.

Development

Mammalian stem cells differentiate into several kinds of blood cell within the bone marrow. This process is called haematopoiesis. All lymphocytes originate, during this process, from a common lymphoid progenitor before differentiating into their distinct lymphocyte types. The differentiation of lymphocytes follows various pathways in a hierarchical fashion as well as in a more plastic fashion. The formation of lymphocytes is known as lymphopoiesis. B cells mature into B lymphocytes in the bursa equivalent, which in humans is the GALT, which is thought to be located in the Peyer's patches of the intestine, while T cells migrate to and mature in a distinct organ, called the thymus. Following maturation, the lymphocytes enter the circulation and peripheral lymphoid organs (e.g. the spleen and lymph nodes) where they survey for invading pathogens and/or tumor cells.

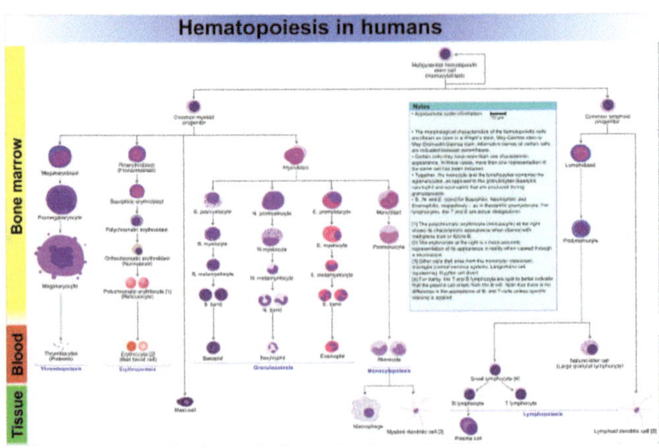

Development of blood cells

The lymphocytes involved in adaptive immunity (i.e. B and T cells) differentiate further after exposure to an antigen; they form effector and memory lymphocytes. Effector lymphocytes function to eliminate the antigen, either by releasing antibodies (in the case of B cells), cytotoxic granules (cytotoxic T cells) or by signaling to other cells of the immune system (helper T cells). Memory T cells remain in the peripheral tissues and circulation for an extended time ready to respond to the same antigen upon future exposure; they live weeks to several years to a whole lifetime, which is very long compared to other leukocytes.

Characteristics

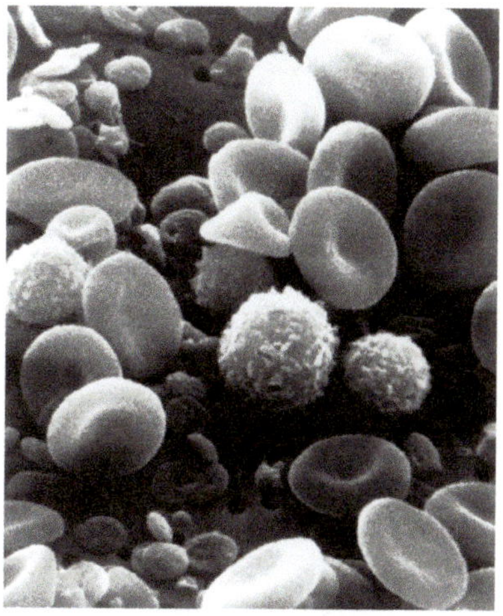

A scanning electron microscope image of normal circulating human blood showing red blood cells, several types of white blood cells including lymphocytes, a monocyte, a neutrophil and many small disc-shaped platelets.

Microscopically, in a Wright's stained peripheral blood smear, a normal lymphocyte has a large, dark-staining nucleus with little to no eosinophilic cytoplasm. In normal situations, the coarse, dense nucleus of a lymphocyte is approximately the size of a red blood cell (about 7 µm in diameter). Some lymphocytes show a clear perinuclear zone (or halo) around the nucleus or could exhibit a small clear zone to one side of the nucleus. Polyribosomes are a prominent feature in the lymphocytes and can be viewed with an electron microscope. The ribosomes are involved in protein synthesis, allowing the generation of large quantities of cytokines and immunoglobulins by these cells.

It is impossible to distinguish between T cells and B cells in a peripheral blood smear. Normally, flow cytometry testing is used for specific lymphocyte population counts. This can be used to determine the percentage of lymphocytes that contain a particular combination of specific cell surface proteins, such as immunoglobulins or cluster of differentiation (CD) markers or that produce particular proteins (for example, cytokines using intracellular cytokine staining (ICCS)). In order to study the function of a lymphocyte by virtue of the proteins it generates, other scientific techniques like the ELISPOT or secretion assay techniques can be used.

Typical recognition markers for lymphocytes			
Class	**Function**	**Proportion**	**Phenotypic marker(s)**
Natural killer cells	Lysis of virally infected cells and tumour cells	7% (2–13%)	CD16 CD56 but not CD3
T helper cells	Release cytokines and growth factors that regulate other immune cells	46% (28–59%)	TCRαβ, CD3 and CD4
Cytotoxic T cells	Lysis of virally infected cells, tumour cells and allografts	19% (13–32%)	TCRαβ, CD3 and CD8
Gamma delta T cells	Immunoregulation and cytotoxicity	5% (2–8%)	TCRγδ and CD3
B cells	Secretion of antibodies	23% (18–47%)	MHC class II, CD19 and CD21

In the circulatory system, they move from lymph node to lymph node. This contrasts with macrophages, which are rather stationary in the nodes.

Lymphocytes and disease

A lymphocyte count is usually part of a peripheral complete blood cell count and is expressed as the percentage of lymphocytes to the total number of white blood cells counted.

A general increase in the number of lymphocytes is known as lymphocytosis, whereas a decrease is known as lymphocytopenia.

High

An increase in lymphocyte concentration is usually a sign of a viral infection (in some rare case, leukemias are found through an abnormally raised lymphocyte count in an otherwise normal person). A high lymphocyte count with a low neutrophil count might be caused by lymphoma. Pertussis toxin (PTx) of *Bordetella pertussis*, formerly known as lymphocytosis-promoting factor, causes a decrease in the entry of lymphocytes into lymph nodes, which can lead to a condition known as lymphocytosis, with a complete lymphocyte count of over 4000 per μl in adults or over 8000 per μl in children. This is unique in that many bacterial infections illustrate neutrophil-predominance instead.

Low

A low normal to low absolute lymphocyte concentration is associated with increased rates of infection after surgery or trauma.

One basis for low T cell lymphocytes occurs when the human immunodeficiency virus (HIV) infects and destroys T cells (specifically, the $CD4^+$ subgroup of T lymphocytes). Without the key defense that these T cells provide, the body becomes susceptible to opportunistic infections that otherwise would not affect healthy people. The extent of HIV progression is typically determined by measuring the percentage of CD4$^+$ T cells in the patient's blood – HIV ultimately progresses to acquired immune deficiency syndrome (AIDS). The effects of other viruses or lymphocyte disorders can also often be estimated by counting the numbers of lymphocytes present in the blood.

Tumor-infiltrating Lymphocytes

In some cancers, such as melanoma and colorectal cancer, lymphocytes can migrate into and attack the tumor. This can sometimes lead to regression of the primary tumor.

Blood Content

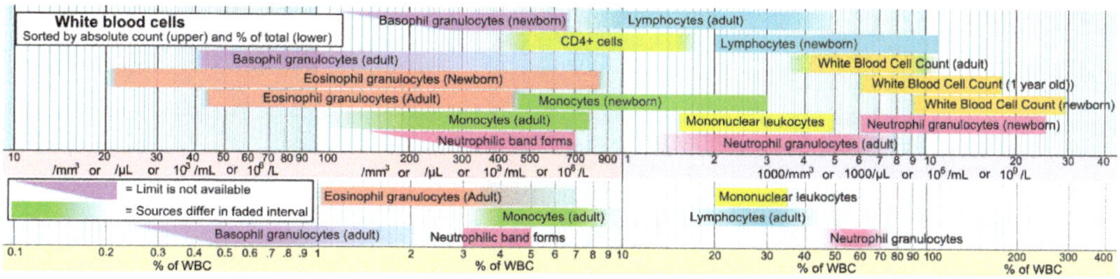

Reference ranges for blood tests of white blood cells, comparing lymphocyte amount (shown in light blue) with other cells.

T Cell

A T cell, or T lymphocyte, is a type of lymphocyte (a subtype of white blood cell) that plays a central role in cell-mediated immunity. T cells can be distinguished from other lymphocytes, such as B cells and natural killer cells, by the presence of a T-cell receptor on the cell surface. They are called *T cells* because they mature in the thymus from thymocytes (although some also mature in the tonsils). The several subsets of T cells each have a distinct function. The majority of human T cells rearrange their alpha and beta chains on the cell receptor and are termed alpha beta T cells (αβ T cells) and are part of the adaptive immune system. Specialized gamma delta T cells, (a small minority of T cells in the human body, more frequent in ruminants), have invariant T cell receptors with limited diversity, that can effectively present antigens to other T cells and are considered to be part of the innate immune system.

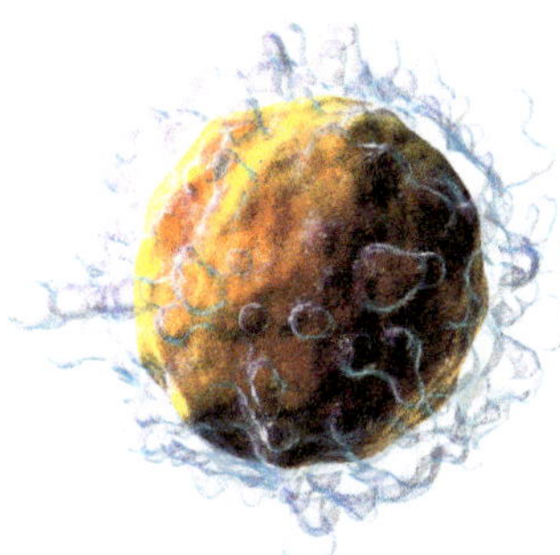

3D rendering of a T cell

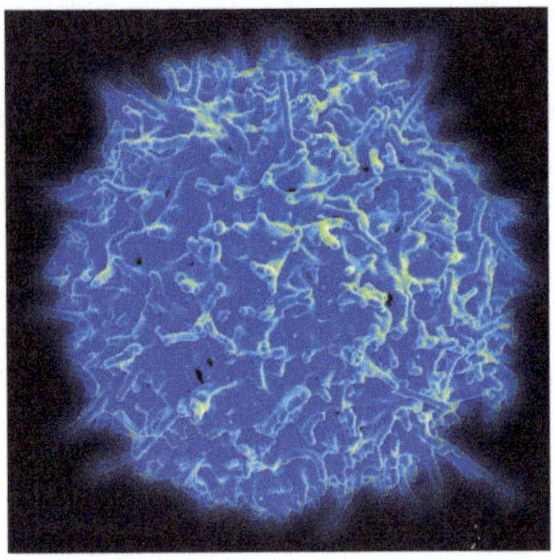

Scanning electron micrograph of a human T cell

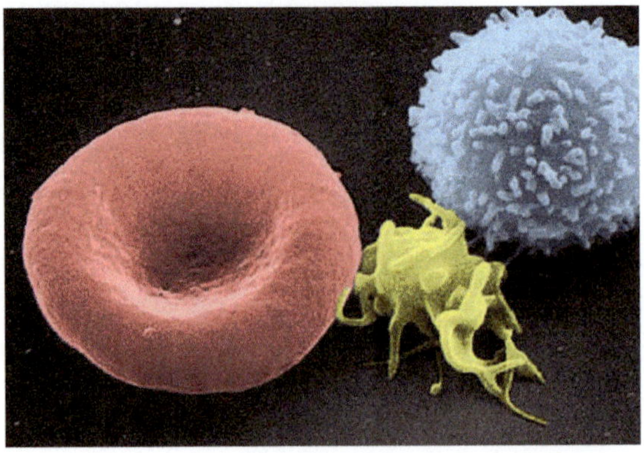

Scanning electron micrograph of T lymphocyte (right), a platelet (center) and a red blood cell (left)

Types

Effector

The category of effector T cell is a broad one that includes various T cell types that actively respond to a stimulus, such as co-stimulation. This includes helper, killer, regulatory, and potentially other T cell types.

Helper

T helper cells (T_H cells) assist other white blood cells in immunologic processes, including maturation of B cells into plasma cells and memory B cells, and activation of cytotoxic T cells and macrophages. These cells are also known as $CD4^+$ T cells because they express the CD4 glycoprotein on their surfaces. Helper T cells become activated when they are presented with peptide antigens by MHC class II molecules, which are expressed on the surface of antigen-presenting cells (APCs). Once activated, they divide rapidly and secrete small proteins called cytokines that regulate or assist in the active immune response. These cells can differentiate into one of several subtypes, including T_H1, T_H2, T_H3, T_H17, T_H9, or T_{FH}, which secrete different cytokines to facilitate different types of immune responses. Signalling from the APC directs T cells into particular subtypes.

Cytotoxic (Killer)

Cytotoxic T cells (T_C cells, CTLs, T-killer cells, killer T cells) destroy virus-infected cells and tumor cells, and are also implicated in transplant rejection. These cells are also known as $CD8^+$ T cells since they express the CD8 glycoprotein at their surfaces. These cells recognize their targets by binding to antigen associated with MHC class I molecules, which are present on the surface of all nucleated cells. Through IL-10, adenosine, and other molecules secreted by regulatory T cells, the $CD8^+$ cells can be inactivated to an anergic state, which prevents autoimmune diseases.

Memory

Memory T cells are a subset of antigen-specific T cells that persist long-term after an infection has resolved. They quickly expand to large numbers of effector T cells upon re-exposure to their cognate antigen, thus providing the immune system with "memory" against past infections.

Memory cells may be either $CD4^+$ or $CD8^+$. Memory T cells typically express the cell surface protein CD45RO.

Memory T cells comprise three subtypes:

- central memory T cells (T_{CM} cells),
- effector memory T cells (T_{EM} cells and T_{EMRA} cells) and
- resident memory T cells (T_{RM}).

Regulatory (Suppressor)

Regulatory T cells (suppressor T cells) are crucial for the maintenance of immunological tolerance. Their major role is to shut down T cell-mediated immunity toward the end of an immune reaction and to suppress autoreactive T cells that escaped the process of negative selection in the thymus. Suppressor T cells along with Helper T cells can collectively be called Regulatory T cells due to their regulatory functions.

Two major classes of $CD4^+$ T_{reg} cells have been described — $FOXP3^+$ T_{reg} cells and $FOXP3^-$ T_{reg} cells.

Regulatory T cells can develop either during normal development in the thymus, and are then known as thymic Treg cells, or can be induced peripherally and are called peripherally derived Treg cells. These two subsets were previously called "naturally occurring", and "adaptive" or "induced", respectively. Both subsets require the expression of the transcription factor FOXP3 which can be used to identify the cells. Mutations of the *FOXP3* gene can prevent regulatory T cell development, causing the fatal autoimmune disease IPEX.

Several other types of T cell have suppressive activity, but do not express FOXP3. These include Tr1 cells and Th3 cells, which are thought to originate during an immune response and act by producing suppressive molecules. Tr1 cells are associated with IL-10, and Th3 cells are associated with TGF-beta. Recently, Treg17 cells have been added to this list.

Natural Killer T Cell

Natural killer T cells bridge the adaptive immune system with the innate immune system. Unlike conventional T cells that recognize peptide antigens presented by major histocompatibility complex (MHC) molecules, NKT cells recognize glycolipid antigen presented by a molecule called CD1d. Once activated, these cells can perform functions ascribed to both T_h and T_c cells (i.e., cytokine production and release of cytolytic/cell killing molecules). They are also able to recognize and eliminate some tumor cells and cells infected with herpes viruses.

Mucosal Associated Invariant

Mucosal associated invariant T cells (MAITs) are a special type of T cell recognised since about 2009.

Gamma Delta T Cells

Gamma delta T cells (γδ T cells) represent a small subset of T cells that possess a distinct T cell receptor (TCR) on their surfaces. A majority of T cells have a TCR composed of two glycoprotein chains called α- and β- TCR chains. However, in γδ T cells, the TCR is made up of one γ-chain and one δ-chain. This group of T cells is much less common in humans and mice (about 2% of total T cells); and are found mostly in the gut mucosa, within a population of lymphocytes known as intraepithelial lymphocytes. In rabbits, sheep, and chickens, the number of γδ T cells can be as high as 60% of total T cells. The antigenic molecules that activate γδ T cells are still widely unknown. However, γδ T cells are not MHC-restricted and seem to be able to recognize whole proteins rather than requiring peptides to be presented by MHC molecules on APCs. Some murine γδ T cells recognize MHC class IB molecules, though. Human Vγ9/Vδ2 T cells, which constitute the major γδ T cell population in peripheral blood, are unique in that they specifically and rapidly respond to a set of nonpeptidic phosphorylated isoprenoid precursors, collectively named phosphoantigens, which are produced by virtually all living cells. The most common phosphoantigens from animal and human cells (including cancer cells) are isopentenyl pyrophosphate (IPP) and its isomer dimethylallyl pyrophosphate (DMPP). Many microbes produce the highly active compound hydroxy-DMAPP (HMB-PP) and corresponding mononucleotide conjugates, in addition to IPP and DMAPP. Plant cells produce both types of phosphoantigens. Drugs activating human Vγ9/Vδ2 T cells comprise synthetic phosphoantigens and aminobisphosphonates, which upregulate endogenous IPP/DMAPP.

Development in the Thymus

All T cells originate from haematopoietic stem cells in the bone marrow. Haematopoietic progenitors (lymphoid progenitor cells) from haematopoietic stem cells populate the thymus and expand by cell division to generate a large population of immature thymocytes. The earliest thymocytes express neither CD4 nor CD8, and are therefore classed as double-negative ($CD4^-CD8^-$) cells. As they progress through their development, they become double-positive thymocytes ($CD4^+CD8^+$), and finally mature to *single-positive* ($CD4^+CD8^-$ or $CD4^-CD8^+$) thymocytes that are then released from the thymus to peripheral tissues. There is some evidence of double-positive T-cells in the periphery, though their prevalence and function is uncertain.

About 98% of thymocytes die during the development processes in the thymus by failing either positive selection or negative selection, whereas the other 2% survive and leave the thymus to become mature immunocompetent T cells. Increasing evidence indicates microRNAs, which are small noncoding regulatory RNAs, could impact the clonal selection process during thymic development. For example, miR-181a was found to play a role in the positive selection of T lymphocytes.

The thymus contributes fewer cells as a person ages. As the thymus shrinks by about 3% a year throughout middle age, a corresponding fall in the thymic production of naïve T cells occurs, leaving peripheral T cell expansion to play a greater role in protecting older subjects.

Beta Selection

Common lymphoid precursor cells that migrate to the thymus become known as T-cell precursors (or thymocytes) and do not express a T cell receptor. Broadly speaking, the double negative (DN) stage is focused on producing a functional β-chain whereas the double positive (DP) stage is focused on producing a functional α-chain, ultimately producing a functional αβ T cell receptor. As the developing thymocyte progresses through the four DN stages (DN1, DN2, DN3, and DN4), the T cell expresses an invariant α-chain but rearranges the β-chain locus. If the rearranged β-chain successfully pairs with the invariant α-chain, signals are produced which cease rearrangement of the β-chain (and silence the alternate allele) and result in proliferation of the cell. Although these signals require this pre-TCR at the cell surface, they are independent of ligand binding to the pre-TCR. These thymocytes will then express both CD4 and CD8 and progresses to the double positive (DP) stage where selection of the α-chain takes place. If a rearranged β-chain does not lead to any signalling (e.g. as a result of an inability to pair with the invariant α-chain), the cell may die by neglect (lack of signalling).

Positive Selection

Positive selection "selects for" T cells capable of interacting with MHC. Positive selection involves the production of a signal by double-positive precursors that express either MHC Class I or II restricted receptors. The signal produced by these thymocytes result in RAG gene repression, long-term survival and migration into the medulla, as well as differentiation into mature T cells. The process of positive selection takes a number of days.

Double-positive thymocytes ($CD4^+/CD8^+$) move deep into the thymic cortex, where they are presented with self-antigens. These self-antigens are expressed by thymic cortical epithelial cells on MHC molecules on the surface of cortical epithelial cells. Only those thymocytes that interact with MHC-I or MHC-II appropriately (i.e., not too strongly or too weakly) will receive a vital "survival signal". All that cannot (i.e., if they do not interact strongly enough, or if they bind too strongly) will die by "death by neglect" (no survival signal). This process ensures that the selected T-cells will have an MHC affinity that can serve useful functions in the body (i.e., the cells must be able to interact with MHC and peptide complexes to effect immune responses). The vast majority of all thymocytes end up dying during this process.

A thymocyte's fate is determined during positive selection. Double-positive cells ($CD4^+/CD8^+$) that interact well with MHC class II molecules will eventually become $CD4^+$ cells, whereas thymocytes that interact well with MHC class I molecules mature into $CD8^+$ cells. A T cell becomes a $CD4^+$ cell by down-regulating expression of its CD8 cell surface receptors. If the cell does not lose its signal, it will continue downregulating CD8 and become a $CD4^+$, single positive cell. But, if there is a signal interruption, the cell stops downregulating CD8 and switches over to downregulating CD4 molecules, instead, eventually becoming a $CD8^+$, single positive cell.

This process does not remove thymocytes that may cause autoimmunity. The potentially autoimmune cells are removed by the process of negative selection, which occurs in the thymic medulla (discussed below).

Negative Selection

Negative selection removes thymocytes that are capable of strongly binding with "self" MHC peptides. Thymocytes that survive positive selection migrate towards the boundary of the cortex and medulla in the thymus. While in the medulla, they are again presented with a self-antigen presented on the MHC complex of medullary thymic epithelial cells (mTECs). mTECs must be $AIRE^+$ to properly express self-antigens from all tissues of the body on their MHC class I peptides. Some mTECs are phagocytosed by thymic dendritic cells; this allows for presentation of self-antigens on MHC class II molecules (positively selected $CD4^+$ cells must interact with MHC class II molecules, thus APCs, which possess MHC class II, must be present for $CD4^+$ T-cell negative selection). Thymocytes that interact too strongly with the self-antigen receive an apoptotic signal that leads to cell death. However, some of these cells are selected to become Treg cells. The remaining cells exit the thymus as mature naïve T cells (also known as recent thymic emigrants). This process is an important component of central tolerance and serves to prevent the formation of self-reactive T cells that are capable of inducing autoimmune diseases in the host.

In summary, β-selection is the first checkpoint, where the T cells that are able to form a functional pre-TCR with an invariant alpha chain and a functional beta chain are allowed to continue development in the thymus. Next, positive selection checks that T cells have successfully rearranged their TCRα locus and are capable of recognizing peptide-MHC complexes with appropriate affinity. Negative selection in the medulla then obliterates T cells that bind too strongly to self-antigens expressed on MHC molecules. These selection processes allow for tolerance of self by the immune system. Typical T-cells that leave the thymus (via the cortico-medullarly junction) are self-restricted, self-tolerant, and singly positive.

Activation

Activation of $CD4^+$ T cells occurs through the simultaneous engagement of the T cell receptor and a co-stimulatory molecule (like CD28, or ICOS) on the T cell by the major histocompatibility complex (MHCII) peptide and co-stimulatory molecules on the APC. Both are required for production of an effective immune response; in the absence of co-stimulation, T-cell receptor signalling alone results in anergy. The signalling pathways downstream from co-stimulatory molecules usually engages the PI3K pathway generating PIP3 at the plasma membrane and recruiting PH domain containing signaling molecules like PDK1 that are essential for the activation of PKCθ, and eventual IL-2 production. Optimal $CD8^+$ T cell response relies on $CD4^+$ signalling. $CD4^+$ cells are useful in the initial antigenic activation of naïve CD8 T cells, and sustaining memory $CD8^+$ T cells in the aftermath of an acute infection. Therefore, activation of $CD4^+$ T cells can be beneficial to the action of $CD8^+$ T cells.

The first signal is provided by binding of the T cell receptor to its cognate peptide presented on MHCII on an APC. MHCII is restricted to so-called professional antigen-presenting cells, like dendritic cells, B cells, and macrophages, to name a few. The peptides presented to $CD8^+$ T cells by MHC class I molecules are 8–9 amino acids in length; the peptides presented to $CD4^+$ cells by MHC class II molecules are longer, usually 12–25 amino acids in length, as the ends of the binding cleft of the MHC class II molecule are open.

The second signal comes from co-stimulation, in which surface receptors on the APC are induced by a relatively small number of stimuli, usually products of pathogens, but sometimes breakdown products of cells, such as necrotic-bodies or heat shock proteins. The only co-stimulatory receptor expressed constitutively by naïve T cells is CD28, so co-stimulation for these cells comes from the CD80 and CD86 proteins, which together constitute the B7 protein, (B7.1 and B7.2, respectively) on the APC. Other receptors are expressed upon activation of the T cell, such as OX40 and ICOS, but these largely depend upon CD28 for their expression. The second signal licenses the T cell to respond to an antigen. Without it, the T cell becomes anergic, and it becomes more difficult for it to activate in future. This mechanism prevents inappropriate responses to self, as self-peptides will not usually be presented with suitable co-stimulation. Once a T cell has been appropriately activated (i.e. has received signal one and signal two) it alters its cell surface expression of a variety of proteins. Markers of T cell activation include CD69, CD71 and CD25 (also a marker for Treg cells), and HLA-DR (a marker of human T cell activation). CTLA-4 expression is also up-regulated on activated T cells, which in turn outcompetes CD28 for binding to the B7 proteins. This is a checkpoint mechanism to prevent over activation of the T cell. Activated T cells also change their cell surface glycosylation profile.

The T cell receptor exists as a complex of several proteins. The actual T cell receptor is composed of two separate peptide chains, which are produced from the independent T cell receptor alpha and beta (*TCRα* and *TCRβ*) genes. The other proteins in the complex are the CD3 proteins: CD3εγ and CD3εδ heterodimers and, most important, a CD3ζ homodimer, which has a total of six ITAM motifs. The ITAM motifs on the CD3ζ can be phosphorylated by Lck and in turn recruit ZAP-70. Lck and/or ZAP-70 can also phosphorylate the tyrosines on many other molecules, not least CD28, LAT and SLP-76, which allows the aggregation of signalling complexes around these proteins.

Phosphorylated LAT recruits SLP-76 to the membrane, where it can then bring in PLC-γ, VAV1, Itk and potentially PI3K. PLC-γ cleaves PI(4,5)P2 on the inner leaflet of the membrane to create the active intermediaries diacylglycerol (DAG), inositol-1,4,5-trisphosphate (IP3); PI3K also acts on PIP2, phosphorylating it to produce phosphatidlyinositol-3,4,5-trisphosphate (PIP3). DAG binds and activates some PKCs. Most important in T cells is PKCθ, critical for activating the transcription factors NF-κB and AP-1. IP3 is released from the membrane by PLC-γ and diffuses rapidly to activate calcium channel receptors on the ER, which induces the release of calcium into the cytosol. Low calcium in the endoplasmic reticulum causes STIM1 clustering on the ER membrane and leads to activation of cell membrane CRAC channels that allows additional calcium to flow into the cytosol from the extracellular space. This aggregated cytosolic calcium binds calmodulin, which can then activate calcineurin. Calcineurin, in turn, activates NFAT, which then translocates to the nucleus. NFAT is a transcription factor that activates the transcription of a pleiotropic set of genes, most notable, IL-2, a cytokine that promotes long-term proliferation of activated T cells.

PLCγ can also initiate the NF-κB pathway. DAG activates PKCθ, which then phosphorylates CARMA1, causing it to unfold and function as a scaffold. The cytosolic domains bind an adapter BCL10 via CARD (Caspase activation and recruitment domains) domains; that then binds TRAF6, which is ubiquitinated at K63. This form of ubiquitination does not lead to degradation of target proteins. Rather, it serves to recruit NEMO, IKKα and -β, and TAB1-2/ TAK1. TAK 1 phosphorylates IKK-β, which then phosphorylates IκB allowing for K48 ubiquitination: leads to proteosomal degradation. Rel A and p50 can then enter the nucleus and bind the NF-κB response element. This coupled with NFAT signaling allows for complete activation of the IL-2 gene.

While in most cases activation is dependent on TCR recognition of antigen, alternative pathways for activation have been described. For example, cytotoxic T cells have been shown to become activated when targeted by other CD8 T cells leading to tolerization of the latter.

In spring 2014, the T-Cell Activation in Space (TCAS) experiment was launched to the International Space Station on the SpaceX CRS-3 mission to study how "deficiencies in the human immune system are affected by a microgravity environment"

Antigen Discrimination

A unique feature of T cells is their ability to discriminate between healthy and abnormal (e.g. infected or cancerous) cells in the body. Healthy cells typically express a large number of self derived pMHC on their cell surface and although the T cell antigen receptor can interact with at least a subset of these self pMHC, the T cell generally ignores these healthy cells. However, when these very same cells contain even minute quantities of pathogen derived pMHC, T cells are able to become activated and initiate immune responses. The ability of T cells to ignore healthy cells but respond when these same cells contain pathogen (or cancer) derived pMHC is known as antigen discrimination. The molecular mechanisms that underlie this process are controversial.

Genetic engineering

In 2015, a team of researchers led by Dr. Alexander Marson at the University of California, San Francisco successfully edited the genome of human T cells using a Cas9 ribonucleoprotein delivery method. This advancement has potential for applications in treating "cancer immunotherapies and cell-based therapies for HIV, primary immune deficiencies, and autoimmune diseases".

Disorders

Deficiency

Causes of T cell deficiency include lymphocytopenia of T cells and/or defects on function of individual T cells. Complete insufficiency of T cell function can result from hereditary conditions such as severe combined immunodeficiency (SCID), Omenn syndrome, and cartilage–hair hypoplasia. Causes of partial insufficiencies of T cell function include acquired immune deficiency syndrome (AIDS), and hereditary conditions such as DiGeorge syndrome (DGS), chromosomal breakage syndromes (CBSs), and B-cell and T-cell combined disorders such as ataxia-telangiectasia (AT) and Wiskott–Aldrich syndrome (WAS).

The main pathogens of concern in T cell deficiencies are intracellular pathogens, including *Herpes simplex virus*, *Mycobacterium* and *Listeria*. Also, fungal infections are also more common and severe in T cell deficiencies.

Cancer

Cancer of T cells is termed T-cell lymphoma, and accounts for perhaps one in ten cases of non-Hodgkin lymphoma. The main forms of T cell lymphoma are:

- Extranodal T cell lymphoma
- Cutaneous T cell lymphomas: Sézary syndrome and Mycosis fungoides

- Anaplastic large cell lymphoma
- Angioimmunoblastic T cell lymphoma

T-cell Exhaustion

T-cell exhaustion is the progressive loss of T-cell function. It can occur during sepsis and after other acute or chronic infections.

T-cell exhaustion is mediated by several inhibitory receptors including programmed cell death protein 1 (PD1), TIM3, and lymphocyte activation gene 3 protein (LAG3).

Cytotoxic T Cell

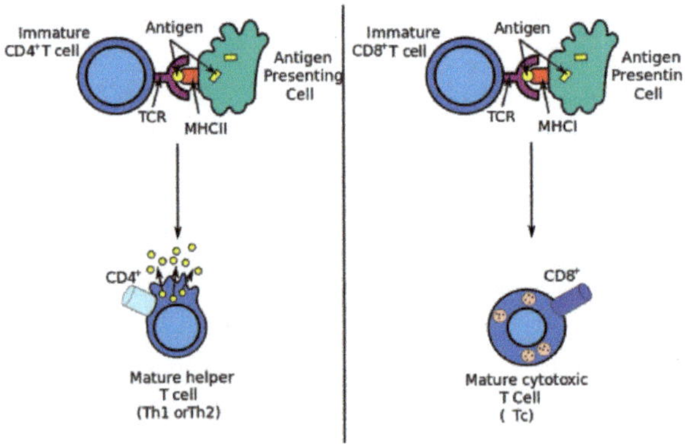

Antigen presentation stimulates T cells to become either "cytotoxic" CD8+ cells or "helper" CD4+ cells.

A cytotoxic T cell (also known as T_C, cytotoxic T lymphocyte, CTL, T-killer cell, cytolytic T cell, CD8+ T-cell or killer T cell) is a T lymphocyte (a type of white blood cell) that kills cancer cells, cells that are infected (particularly with viruses), or cells that are damaged in other ways.

Most cytotoxic T cells express T-cell receptors (TCRs) that can recognize a specific antigen. An antigen is a molecule capable of stimulating an immune response, and is often produced by cancer cells or viruses. Antigens inside a cell are bound to class I MHC molecules, and brought to the surface of the cell by the class I MHC molecule, where they can be recognized by the T cell. If the TCR is specific for that antigen, it binds to the complex of the class I MHC molecule and the antigen, and the T cell destroys the cell.

In order for the TCR to bind to the class I MHC molecule, the former must be accompanied by a glycoprotein called CD8, which binds to the constant portion of the class I MHC molecule. Therefore, these T cells are called CD8+ T cells.

The affinity between CD8 and the MHC molecule keeps the T_C cell and the target cell bound closely together during antigen-specific activation. CD8+ T cells are recognized as T_C cells once they become activated and are generally classified as having a pre-defined cytotoxic role within the immune system. However, CD8+ T cells also have the ability to make some cytokines.

Development

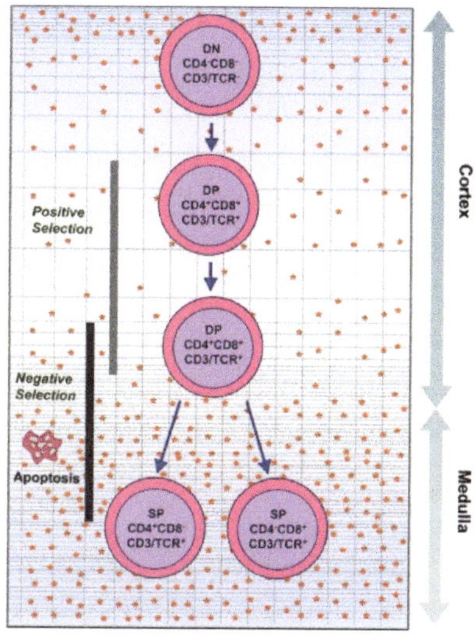

Development of single positive T cells in the thymus

The immune system must recognize millions of potential antigens. There are fewer than 30,000 genes in the human body, so it is impossible to have one gene for every antigen. Instead, the DNA in millions of white blood cells in the bone marrow is shuffled to create cells with unique receptors, each of which can bind to a different antigen. Some receptors bind to tissues in the human body itself, so to prevent the body from attacking itself, those self-reactive white blood cells are destroyed during further development in the thymus.

TCRs have two parts, usually an alpha and a beta chain. (Some TCRs have a gamma and a delta chain.) Hematopoietic stem cells in the bone marrow migrate into the thymus, where they undergo VDJ recombination of their beta-chain TCR DNA to form a developmental form of the TCR protein, known as pre-TCR. If that rearrangement is successful, the cells then rearrange their alpha-chain TCR DNA to create a functional alpha-beta TCR complex. This highly-variable genetic rearrangement product in the TCR genes helps create millions of different T cells with different TCRs, helping the body's immune system respond to virtually any protein of an invader. The vast majority of T cells express alpha-beta TCRs (αβ T cells), but some T cells in epithelial tissues (like the gut) express gamma-delta TCRs (γδ T cells), which recognize non-protein antigens.

T cells with functionally stable TCRs express both the CD4 and CD8 co-receptors and are therefore termed "double-positive" (DP) T cells (CD4+CD8+). The double-positive T cells are exposed to a wide variety of self-antigens in the thymus and undergo two selection criteria:

1. positive selection, in which those double-positive T cells that bind *too weakly* to MHC-presented *self antigens* undergo apoptosis because of their inability to recognize MHC-protein complexes.
2. negative selection, in which those double-positive T cells that bind *too strongly* to MHC-presented *self antigens* undergo apoptosis because they could otherwise become autoreactive, leading to autoimmunity.

Only those T cells that bind to the MHC-self-antigen complexes weakly are positively selected. Those cells that survive positive and negative selection differentiate into single-positive T cells (either CD4+ or CD8+), depending on whether their TCR recognizes an MHC class I-presented antigen (CD8) or an MHC class II-presented antigen (CD4). It is the CD8+ T-cells that will mature and go on to become cytotoxic T cells following their activation with a class I-restricted antigen.

Activation

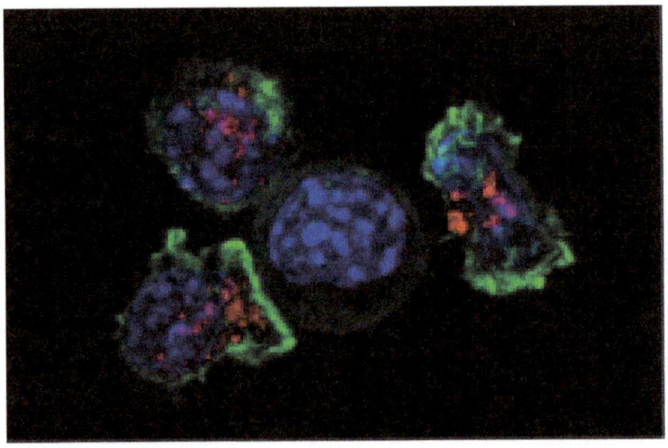

In this immunofluorescence image, a group of killer T cells (outer three) is engaging a cancer cell(centered one). A patch of signaling molecules (pink) that gathers at the site of cell-cell contact indicates that the CTL has identified a target. Lytic granules (red) that contain cytotoxic components then travel along the microtubule cytoskeleton (green) to the contact site and are secreted, thus killing the target.

With an exception of some cell types, such as non-nucleated cells (including erythrocytes), Class I MHC is expressed by all host cells. When these cells are infected with a virus (or another intracellular pathogen), the cells degrade foreign proteins via antigen processing. These result in peptide fragments, some of which are presented by MHC Class I to the T cell antigen receptor (TCR) on CD8+ T cells.

The activation of cytotoxic T cells is dependent on several simultaneous interactions between molecules expressed on the surface of the T cell and molecules on the surface of the antigen-presenting cell (APC). For instance, consider the *two signal model* for T_C cell activation.

Signal	T cell	APC	Description
First Signal	TCR	peptide-bound MHC class I molecule	There is a second interaction between the CD8 coreceptor and the class I MHC molecule to stabilize this signal.
Second Signal	CD28 molecule on the T cell	either CD80 or CD86 (also called B7-1 and B7-2)	CD80 and CD86 are known as *costimulators* for T cell activation. This second signal can be assisted (or replaced) by stimulating the T_C cell with cytokines released from helper T cells.

A simple activation of naive $CD8^+$ T cells requires the interaction with professional antigen-presenting cells, mainly with matured dendritic cells. To generate longlasting memory T cells and to allow repetitive stimulation of cytotoxic T cells, dendritic cells have to interact with both, activated $CD4^+$ helper T cells and $CD8^+$ T cells. During this process, the $CD4^+$ helper T cells "license" the dendritic cells to give a potent activating signal to the naive $CD8^+$ T cells.

While in most cases activation is dependent on TCR recognition of antigen, alternative pathways for activation have been described. For example, cytotoxic T cells have been shown to become activated when targeted by other CD8 T cells leading to tolerization of the latter.

Once activated, the T_C cell undergoes clonal expansion with the help of the cytokine Interleukin-2 (IL-2), which is a growth and differentiation factor for T cells. This increases the number of cells specific for the target antigen that can then travel throughout the body in search of antigen-positive somatic cells.

Effector Functions

When exposed to infected/dysfunctional somatic cells, T_C cells release the cytotoxins perforin, granzymes, and granulysin. Through the action of perforin, granzymes enter the cytoplasm of the target cell and their serine protease function triggers the caspase cascade, which is a series of cysteine proteases that eventually lead to apoptosis (programmed cell death).

A second way to induce apoptosis is via cell-surface interaction between the T_C and the infected cell. When a T_C is activated it starts to express the surface protein FAS ligand (FasL)(Apo1L)(CD95L), which can bind to *Fas* (Apo1)(CD95) molecules expressed on the target cell. However, this Fas-Fas ligand interaction is thought to be more important to the disposal of unwanted T lymphocytes during their development or to the lytic activity of certain T_H cells than it is to the cytolytic activity of T_C effector cells. Engagement of Fas with FasL allows for recruitment of the death-induced signaling complex (DISC). The Fas-associated death domain (FADD) translocates with the DISC, allowing recruitment of procaspases 8 and 10. These caspases then activate the effector caspases 3, 6, and 7, leading to cleavage of death substrates such as lamin A, lamin B1, lamin B2, PARP (poly ADP ribose polymerase), and DNAPK (DNA-activated protein kinase). The final result is apoptosis of the cell that expressed Fas.

Role in Disease Pathogenesis

During hepatitis B virus (HBV) infection cytotoxic T cells play an important pathogenetic role. They contribute to nearly all of the liver injury associated with HBV infection and, by killing infected cells and by producing antiviral cytokines capable of purging HBV from viable hepatocytes, cytotoxic T cells also eliminate the virus. Platelets have been shown to facilitate the accumulation of virus-specific cytotoxic T cells into the infected liver.

Cytotoxic T cells have been implicated in the progression of arthritis: depletion of knee joint cartilage macromolecules such as glycosaminoglycans by cytotoxic T cells and macrophages has been observed in a rat model of the disease.

T Helper Cell

The T helper cells (T_h cells) are a type of T cell that play an important role in the immune system, particularly in the adaptive immune system. They help the activity of other immune cells by releasing T cell cytokines. These cells help suppress or regulate immune responses. They are essential in B cell antibody class switching, in the activation and growth of cytotoxic T cells, and in maximizing bactericidal activity of phagocytes such as macrophages.

Mature T_h cells express the surface protein CD4 and are referred to as $CD4^+$ T cells. Such $CD4^+$ T cells are generally treated as having a pre-defined role as helper T cells within the immune system. For example, when an antigen-presenting cell expresses an antigen on MHC class II, a $CD4^+$ cell will aid those cells through a combination of cell to cell interactions (e.g. CD40 (protein) and CD40L) and through cytokines.

CD154, also called CD40 ligand or CD40L, is a cell surface protein that mediates T cell helper function in a contact-dependent process and is a member of the TNF superfamily of molecules. It binds to CD40 on antigen-presenting cells (APC), which leads to many effects depending on the target cell type. CD154 acts as a costimulatory molecule and is particularly important on a subset of T cells called T follicular helper cells (T_{FH} cells). On T_{FH} cells, CD154 promotes B cell maturation and function by engaging CD40 on the B cell surface and therefore facilitating cell-cell communication. A defect in this gene results in an inability to undergo immunoglobulin class switching and is associated with hyper IgM syndrome. Absence of CD154 also stops the formation of germinal centers and therefore prohibiting antibody affinity maturation, an important process in the adaptive immune system.

The importance of helper T cells can be seen from HIV, a virus that primarily infects $CD4^+$ T cells. In the advanced stages of HIV infection, loss of functional $CD4^+$ T cells leads to the symptomatic stage of infection known as the acquired immunodeficiency syndrome (AIDS). When the HIV virus is detected early in blood or other bodily fluids, continuous therapy can delay the time at which this fall happens. Therapy can also better manage the course of AIDS if and when it occurs. There are other rare disorders such as lymphocytopenia which result in the absence or dysfunction of $CD4^+$ T cells. These disorders produce similar symptoms, many of which are fatal.

Activation of naïve helper T cells

Following T cell development, matured, naïve T cells leave the thymus and begin to spread throughout the body, including the lymph nodes. (Naïve T cells are those T cells that have never been exposed to the antigen that they are programmed to respond to). Like all T cells, they express the T cell receptor-CD3 complex. The T cell receptor (TCR) consists of both constant and variable regions. The variable region determines what antigen the T cell can respond to. $CD4^+$ T cells have TCRs with an affinity for Class II MHC, and CD4 is involved in determining MHC affinity during maturation in the thymus. Class II MHC proteins are generally only found on the surface of specialised antigen-presenting cells (APCs). Specialised antigen presenting cells are primarily dendritic cells, macrophages and B cells, although dendritic cells are the only cell group that expresses MHC Class II constitutively (at all times). Some APCs also bind native (or unprocessed) antigens to their surface, such as follicular dendritic cells, but unprocessed antigens do not interact with T cells and are not involved in their activation. The antigens that bind to MHC proteins are always short peptides, 8-10 amino acids long for MHC Class I, and up to 25 or so for MHC Class II.

Recognition (Signal 1)

During an immune response, professional antigen-presenting cells (APCs) endocytose foreign material (typically bacteria or viruses), which undergoes processing, then travel from the infection site to the lymph nodes. Once at the lymph nodes, the APC begin to present antigen peptides that are bound to Class II MHC, allowing $CD4^+$ T cells that express the specific TCRs against the peptide/MHC complex to activate.

When a T_h cell encounters and recognises the antigen on an APC, the TCR-CD3 complex binds strongly to the peptide-MHC complex present on the surface of professional APCs. CD4, a co-receptor of the TCR complex, also binds to a different section of the MHC molecule. These interactions bring these proteins closer together, allowing the intracellular kinases present on the TCR, CD3 and CD4 proteins to activate each other via phosphorylation. With the assistance of a phosphatase present on the intracellular section of CD45 (common leukocyte antigen), these molecules activate major T_h cell intracellular pathways. These active pathways are known as Signal 1 of T cell activation, as it is the first and primary pro-activation signal in a T_h cell. Upon subsequent encounters with a given antigen, memory T cells are re-activated using the same TCR pathways.

The binding of the antigen-MHC to the TCR complex and CD4 may also help the APC and the T_h cell adhere during T_h cell activation, but the integrin protein LFA-1 on the T cell and ICAM on the APC are the primary molecules of adhesion in this cell interaction.

It is unknown what role the relatively bulky extracellular region of CD45 plays during cell interactions, but CD45 has various isoforms that change in size depending on the T_h cell's activation and maturation status. For example, CD45 shortens in length following T_h activation (CD45RA$^+$ to CD45RO$^+$), but whether this change in length influences activation is unknown. It has been proposed that the larger CD45RA+ may decrease the accessibility of the T cell receptor for the antigen-MHC molecule, thereby necessitating an increase in the affinity (and specificity) of the T cell for activation. Once the activation has occurred however, CD45 shortens, allowing easier interactions and activation as an effector T helper cell.

Verification (signal 2)

Having received the first TCR/CD3 signal, the naïve T cell must activate a second independent biochemical pathway, known as Signal 2. This verification step is a protective measure to ensure that a T cell is responding to a foreign antigen. If this second signal is not present during initial antigen exposure, the T cell presumes that it is auto-reactive. This results in the cell becoming anergic (anergy is generated from the unprotected biochemical changes of Signal 1). Anergic cells will not respond to any antigen in the future, even if both signals are present later on. These cells are generally believed to circulate throughout the body with no value until they undergo apoptosis.

The second signal involves an interaction between CD28 on the CD4$^+$ T cell and the proteins CD80 (B7.1) or CD86 (B7.2) on the professional APCs. Both CD80 and CD86 activate the CD28 receptor. These proteins are also known as co-stimulatory molecules.

Although the verification stage is necessary for the activation of naïve helper T cells, the importance of this stage is best demonstrated during the similar activation mechanism of CD8$^+$ cytotoxic T cells. As naïve CD8$^+$ T cells have no true bias towards foreign sources, these T cells must rely on the activation of CD28 for confirmation that they recognise a foreign antigen (as CD80/CD86 is only expressed by active APC's). CD28 plays an important role in decreasing the risk of T cell auto-immunity against host antigens.

Once the naïve T cell has both pathways activated, the biochemical changes induced by Signal 1 are altered, allowing the cell to activate instead of anergise. The second signal is then obsolete; only the first signal is necessary for future activation. This is also true for memory T cells, which is one example of learned immunity. Faster responses occur upon reinfection because memory T cells have already undergone confirmation and can produce effector cells much sooner.

Proliferation

Once the two-signal activation is complete the T helper cell (T_h) then allows itself to proliferate. It achieves this by releasing a potent T cell growth factor called interleukin 2 (IL-2) which acts upon itself in an autocrine fashion. Activated T cells also produce the alpha sub-unit of the IL-2 receptor (CD25 or IL-2R), enabling a fully functional receptor that can bind with IL-2, which in turn activates the T cell's proliferation pathways.

The autocrine or paracrine secretion of IL-2 can bind to that same T_h cell or neighboring T_h's via the IL-2R thus driving proliferation and clonal expansion. The T_h cells receiving both signals of activation and proliferation will then become T_h0 cells (T helper 0) cell that secrete IL-2, IL-4 and interferon gamma (IFN-γ). The T_h0 cells will then differentiate into T_h1 or T_h2 cells depending on cytokine environment. IFN-γ drives T_h1 cell production while IL-10 and IL-4 inhibit T_h1 cell production. Conversely, IL-4 drives T_h2 cell production and IFN-γ inhibits T_h2 cells. It should be noted that these cytokines are pleiotropic and carry out many other functions of the immune response.

Maturation

After many cell generations, the T_h cell's progenitors differentiate into effector T_h cells, memory T_h cells, and regulatory T_h cells.

- Effector T_h cells secrete cytokines, proteins or peptides that stimulate or interact with other leukocytes, including T_h cells.
- Memory T_h cells retain the antigen affinity of the originally activated T cell, and are used to act as later effector cells during a second immune response (e.g. if there is re-infection of the host at a later stage).
- Regulatory T cells do not promote immune function, but act to decrease it instead. Despite their low numbers during an infection, these cells are believed to play an important role in the self-limitation of the immune system; they have been shown to prevent the development of various autoimmune diseases.

Effector Function

In 1991, three groups reported discovering CD154, which is the molecular basis of T cell helper function. Seth Lederman at Columbia University generated an murine monoclonal antibody, 5c8 that inhibited contact-dependent T cell helper function in human cells which characterized the 32 kDa surface protein transiently expressed on CD4+ T cells. Richard Armitage at Immunex cloned a cDNA encoding CD154 by screening an expression library with CD40-Ig. Randolph Noelle at Dartmouth Medical School generated an antibody that bound a 39 kDa protein on murine T cells and inhibited helper function.

Determination of the Effector T Cell response

Helper T cells are capable of influencing a variety of immune cells, and the T cell response generated (including the extracellular signals such as cytokines) can be essential for a successful outcome from infection. In order to be effective, helper T cells must determine which cytokines will allow the immune system to be most useful or beneficial for the host. Understanding exactly how helper T cells respond to immune challenges is currently of major interest in immunology, because such knowledge may be very useful in the treatment of disease and in increasing the effectiveness of vaccination.

Th1/Th2 Model for Helper T Cells

Proliferating helper T cells that develop into effector T cells differentiate into two major subtypes of cells known as T_h1 and T_h2 cells (also known as Type 1 and Type 2 helper T cells, respectively).

T_h1 helper cells are the host immunity effectors against intracellular bacteria and protozoa. They are triggered by IL-12, IL-2 and their effector cytokine is IFN-γ. The main effector cells of T_h1 immunity are macrophages as well as CD8 T cells, IgG B cells, and IFN-γ CD4 T cells. The key T_h1 transcription factors are STAT4 and T-bet. IFN-γ secreted by CD4 T cells can activate macrophages to phagocytose and digest intracellular bacteria and protozoa. In addition, IFN-γ can activate iNOS to produce NOx free radicals to directly kill intracellular bacteria and protozoa. T_h1 overactivation against autoantigens will cause Type 4 delayed-type hypersensitivity. Tuberculin reaction or Type 1 diabetes belong to this category of autoimmunity.

T_h2 helper cells are the host immunity effectors against extracellular parasites including helminths. They are triggered by IL-4 and their effector cytokines are IL-4, IL-5, IL-9, IL-10 and IL-13. The main effector cells are eosinophils, basophils, and mast cells as well as B cells, and IL-4/IL-5 CD4 T cells. The key T_h2 transcription factors are STAT6 and GATA3. IL-4 is the positive feedback cytokine for Th2 cells differentiation. Besides, IL-4 stimulates B-cells to produce IgE antibodies, which in turn stimulate mast cells to release histamine, serotonin, and leukotriene to cause broncho-constriction, intestinal peristalsis, gastric fluid acidification to expel helminths. IL-5 from CD4 T cells will activate eosinophils to attack helminths. IL-10 suppresses Th1 cells differentiation and function of dendritic cells. T_h2 overactivation against autoantigen will cause Type1 IgE-mediated allergy and hypersensitivity. Allergic rhinitis, atopic dermatitis, and asthma belong to this category of autoimmunity. In addition to expressing different cytokines, Th2 cells also differ from Th1 cells in their cell surface glycans (oligosaccharides), which makes them less susceptible to some inducers of cell death.

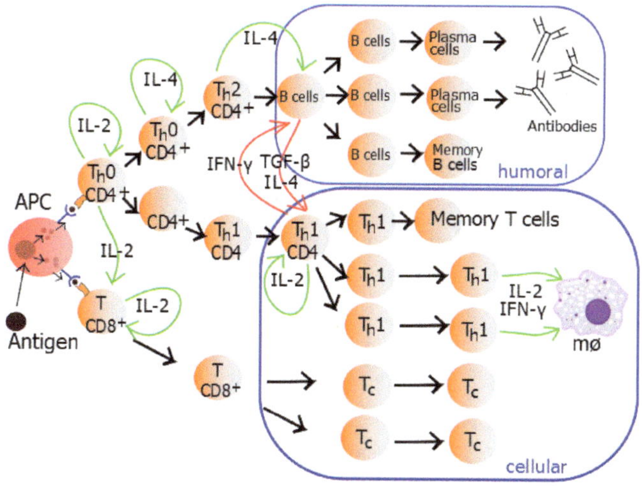

T_h1/T_h2 Model for helper T cells. An antigen is ingested and processed by an APC. It presents fragments from it to T cells. The upper, T_h0, is a T helper cell. The fragment is presented to it by MHC2. IFN-γ, interferon γ; TGF-β, transforming growth factor β; mø, macrophage; IL-2, interleukin 2; IL-4, interleukin 4

Th1/Th2 dichotomy		
	Type 1/ T_h1	**Type 2/ T_h2**
Main partner cell type	Macrophage, CD8+ T cell	B-cell, eosinophil, mast cell
Cytokines produced	interferon-γ and TNF-β. Interleukin-2 interleukin-10 production has been reported in activated Th1 cell.	interleukin-4, interleukin-5, interleukin-6, interleukin-9, interleukin-10, interleukin-13
Immune stimulation promoted	Cellular immune system. Maximizes the killing efficacy of the macrophages and the proliferation of cytotoxic CD8+ T cells. Also promotes the production of IgG, an opsonizing antibody.	Humoral immune system. Stimulates B-cells into proliferation, to induce B-cell antibody class switching, and to increase neutralizing antibody production. (IgG, IgM and IgA as well as IgE antibodies)
Other functions	The Type 1 cytokine IFN-γ increases the production of interleukin-12 by dendritic cells and macrophages, and via positive feedback, IL-12 stimulates the production of IFN-γ in helper T cells, thereby promoting the T_h1 profile. IFN-gamma also inhibits the production of cytokines such as interleukin-4, an important cytokine associated with the Type 2 response, and thus it also acts to preserve its own response.	The Type 2 response promotes its own profile using two different cytokines. Interleukin-4 acts on helper T cells to promote the production of T_h2 cytokines (including itself; it is auto-regulatory), while interleukin-10 (IL-10) inhibits a variety of cytokines including interleukin-2 and IFN-γ in helper T cells and IL-12 in dendritic cells and macrophages. The combined action of these two cytokines suggests that once the T cell has decided to produce these cytokines, that decision is preserved (and also encourages other T cells to do the same).

While we know about the types of cytokine patterns helper T cells tend to produce, we understand less about how the patterns themselves are decided. Various evidence suggests that the type of APC presenting the antigen to the T cell has a major influence on its profile. Other evidence suggests that the concentration of antigen presented to the T cell during primary activation influences its choice. The presence of some cytokines (such as the ones mentioned above) will also influence the response that will eventually be generated, but our understanding is nowhere near complete.

Th17 Helper Cells

T_h17 helper cells are a subset of T helper cells developmentally distinct from T_h1 and T_h2 lineages producing interleukin 17 (IL-17).

THαβ Helper Cells

THαβ helper cells provide the host immunity against viruses. Their differentiation is triggered by IFN alpha/beta or IL-10. Their key effector cytokine is IL-10. Their main effector cells are NK cells as well as CD8 T cells, IgG B cells, and IL-10 CD4 T cells. The key THαβ transcription factors are STAT1 and STAT3 as well as IRFs. IL-10 from CD4 T cells activate NK cells' ADCC to apoptose virus-infected cells and to induce host as well as viral DNA fragmentation. IFN alpha/beta can suppress transcription to avoid virus replication and transmission. Overactivation of THαβ against autoantigen will cause type 2 antibody-dependent cytotoxic hypersensitivity. Myasthenia gravis or Graves' disease belong to this category.

Limitations to the Th1/Th2 Model

The interactions between cytokines from the T_h1/T_h2 model can be more complicated in some animals. For example, the T_h2 cytokine IL-10 inhibits cytokine production of both T_h subsets in humans. Human IL-10 (hIL-10) suppresses the proliferation and cytokine production of all T cells and the activity of macrophages, but continues to stimulate plasma cells, ensuring that antibody production still occurs. As such, hIL-10 is not believed to truly promote the T_h2 response in humans, but acts to prevent over-stimulation of helper T cells while still maximising the production of antibodies.

There are also other types of T cells that can influence the expression and activation of helper T cells, such as natural regulatory T cells, along with less common cytokine profiles such as the T_h3 subset of helper T cells. Terms such as "regulatory" and "suppression" have become ambiguous after the discovery that helper $CD4^+$ T cells are also capable of regulating (and suppressing) their own responses outside of dedicated regulatory T cells.

One major difference between regulatory T cells and effector T cells is that regulatory T cells typically serve to modulate and deactivate the immune response, while effector T cell groups usually begin with immune-promoting cytokines and then switch to inhibitory cytokines later in their life cycle. The latter is a feature of T_h3 cells, which transform into a regulatory subset after its initial activation and cytokine production.

Both regulatory T cells and T_h3 cells produce the cytokine transforming growth factor-beta (TGF-β) and IL-10. Both cytokines are inhibitory to helper T cells; TGF-β suppresses the activity of most of the immune system. There is evidence to suggest that TGF-β may not suppress activated Th2 cells as effectively as it might suppress naive cells, but it is not typically considered a Th2 cytokine.

The characterisation of another novel T helper subtype, T helper 17 cells (T_h17) has cast further doubt on the basic T_h1/T_h2 model. These IL-17 producing cells were initially described as a pathogenic population implicated in autoimmunity but are now thought to have their own distinct effector and regulatory functions. Of note, recent evidence suggest that functional plasticity is an intrinsic capacity of T helper cells. Indeed, a study in mice demonstrated that T_h17 cells transform into T_h1 cells *in vivo*. A subsequent study furthermore showed that extensive T helper cell plasticity is also prominent in man.

Many of the cytokines in this article are also expressed by other immune cells, and it is becoming clear that while the original T_h1/T_h2 model is enlightening and gives insight into the functions of helper T cells, it is far too simple to define its entire role or actions. Some immunologists question the model completely, as some *in vivo* studies suggest that individual helper T cells usually do not match the specific cytokine profiles of the T_h model, and many cells express cytokines from both profiles. That said, the T_h model has still played an important part in developing our understanding of the roles and behaviour of helper T cells and the cytokines they produce during an immune response.

Recent scientific studies by Stockinger et al. revealed that another T helper subset may exist. Th9 cells are claimed to be an IL9 (interleukin 9)–producing T cell subset focused on defending helminth infections.

Role of Helper T Cells in Disease

Considering the diverse and important role helper T cells play in the immune system, it is not surprising that these cells often influence the immune response against disease. They also appear to make occasional mistakes, or generate responses that would be politely considered non-beneficial. In the worst-case scenario, the helper T cell response could lead to a disaster and the fatality of the host. Fortunately this is a very rare occurrence.

Helper T cells and Hypersensitivity

The immune system must achieve a balance of sensitivity in order to respond to foreign antigens without responding to the antigens of the host itself. When the immune system responds to very low levels of antigen that it usually shouldn't respond to, a hypersensitivity response occurs. Hypersensitivity is believed to be the cause of allergy and some auto-immune disease.

Hypersensitivity reactions can be divided into four types:

- Type 1 hypersensitivity includes common immune disorders such as asthma, allergic rhinitis (hay fever), eczema, urticaria (hives) and anaphylaxis. These reactions all involve IgE antibodies, which require a T_h2 response during helper T cell development. Preventive treatments, such as corticosteroids and montelukast, focus on suppressing mast cells or other allergic cells; T cells do not play a primary role during the actual inflammatory response. It's important to note that the numeral allocation of hypersensitivity "types" does not correlate (and is completely unrelated) to the "response" in the T_h model.
- Type 2 and Type 3 hypersensitivity both involve complications from auto-immune or low affinity antibodies. In both of these reactions, T cells may play an accomplice role in generating these auto-specific antibodies, although some of these reactions under Type 2 hypersensitivity would be considered normal in a healthy immune system (for example, Rhesus factor reactions during childbirth is a normal immune response against child antigens). The understanding of the role of helper T cells in these responses is limited but it is generally thought that T_h2 cytokines would promote such disorders. For example, studies have suggested that lupus (SLE) and other auto-immune diseases of similar nature can be linked to the production of T_h2 cytokines.
- Type 4 hypersensitivity, also known as delayed type hypersensitivity, are caused via the over-stimulation of immune cells, commonly lymphocytes and macrophages, resulting in chronic inflammation and cytokine release. Antibodies do not play a direct role in this allergy type. T cells play an important role in this hypersensitivity, as they activate against the stimulus itself and promote the activation of other cells; particularly macrophages via T_h1 cytokines.

Other cellular hypersensitivities include cytotoxic T cell mediated auto-immune disease, and a similar phenomenon; transplant rejection. Helper T cells are required to fuel the development of these diseases. In order to create sufficient auto-reactive killer T cells, interleukin-2 must be produced, and this is supplied by $CD4^+$ T cells. $CD4^+$ T cells can also stimulate cells such as natural killer cells and macrophages via cytokines such as interferon-gamma, encouraging these cytotoxic cells to kill host cells in certain circumstances.

The mechanism that killer T cells use during auto-immunity is almost identical to their response against viruses, and some viruses have been accused of causing auto-immune diseases such as Type 1 Diabetes mellitus. Cellular auto-immune disease occurs because the host antigen recognition systems fail, and the immune system believes, by mistake, that a host antigen is foreign. As a result, the $CD8^+$ T cells treat the host cell presenting that antigen as infected, and go on to destroy all host cells (or in the case of transplant rejection, transplant organ) that express that antigen.

Many auto-immune diseases are more complex. A well-known example is rheumatoid arthritis, where both antibodies and immune cells are known to play a role in the pathology. Generally the immunology of most auto-immune diseases is not well understood.

HIV Infection

Perhaps the best example of the importance of $CD4^+$ T cells is demonstrated with human immunodeficiency virus (HIV) infection. HIV mainly targets lymphoid $CD4^+$ T cells, but can infect other cells that express CD4 such as macrophages and dendritic cells (both groups express CD4 at low levels).

It has been proposed that during the non-symptomatic phase of HIV infection, the virus has a relatively low affinity towards T cells (and has a higher affinity for macrophages), resulting in a slow kill rate of $CD4^+$ T cells by the immune system. This is initially compensated for via the production of new helper T cells from the thymus (originally from the bone marrow). Once the virus becomes lymphotropic (or T-tropic) however, it begins to infect $CD4^+$ T cells far more efficiently (likely due to a change in the co-receptors it binds to during infection), and the immune system is overwhelmed. Of note, recent studies suggest that only ~5% of the lymphoid-derived CD4 T cells targeted by HIV are permissive and become productively infected with the virus. More than 95% of the CD4 T cells that die are resting and are unable to support productive infection. These cells undergo abortive infection with HIV. Cell death is triggered when the host cell detects HIV foreign DNA intermediates and initiates a suicidal death pathway in an attempt to protect the host, leading to caspase-1 activation in inflammasomes, thus causing pyroptosis (a highly inflammatory form of programmed cell death).

At this point chronic inflammation ensues, and functional $CD4^+$ T cell levels begin to decrease, eventually to a point where the $CD4^+$ T cell population is too small to recognize the full range of antigens that could potentially be detected. The depletion of CD4 T cells and the development of chronic inflammation are signature processes in HIV pathogenesis that propel progression to acquired immune deficiency syndrome (AIDS). CD4 T cell depleted to the cell count of less than 200cell/μL in blood during AIDS allows various pathogens to escape T cell recognition, thus allowing opportunistic infections that would normally elicit a helper T cell response to bypass the immune system. While these complete bypass situations only occur when the helper T cell response is absolutely necessary for infection clearance, most infections increase in severity and/or duration because the immune system's helper T cells provide less efficient immune response.

Two components of the immune system are particularly affected in AIDS, due to its CD4⁺ T cell dependency:

1. CD8⁺ T cells are not stimulated as effectively during the AIDS stage of HIV infection, making AIDS patients very susceptible to most viruses, including HIV itself. This decline in killing of CD4⁺ T cells results in the virus being produced for a longer period (the infected CD4⁺ T cells are not killed as quickly), increasing the proliferation of the virus, and accelerating the development of the disease.

2. Antibody class switching declines significantly once helper T cell function fails. The immune system loses its ability to improve the affinity of their antibodies, and are unable to generate B cells that can produce antibody groups such as IgG and IgA. These effects are primarily due to the loss of any helper T cell that can interact with the B lymphocyte correctly. Another symptom of AIDS is the reduction in antibody levels due to a decrease in T_h2 cytokines (and less interactions by helper T cells). All of these complications result in an increased susceptibility to aggressive bacterial infections, especially in areas of the body not accessible by IgM antibodies.

If the patient does not respond to (or does not receive) HIV treatment they will succumb usually to either cancers or infections; the immune system finally reaches a point where it is no longer coordinated or stimulated enough to deal with the disease.

Inhibition of CD4 T-cell expansion during HIV infection may occur due to microbial translocation in an IL-10-dependent way. Triggering PD-1 expressed on activated monocytes by its ligand PD-L1, induces IL-10 production which inhibits CD4 T-cell function.

Antigen Presentation

Antigen presentation describes a vital immune process which is essential for T cell immune response triggering. Because T cells do recognise only fragmented antigens displayed on the cell surfaces, antigen processing and presentation must proceed before the antigen fragment bound to MHC complex is transported to the surface of the cell in order to stimulate a particular T cell receptor. After infection with viruses or bacteria, the cells present endogenous or exogenous peptide fragments derived from the pathogen bound to major histocompatibility complex (MHC) molecules on the cell surface. There are two types of MHC molecules which differ in the source of the antigens: MHC class I molecules (MHC-I) bind peptides from the cell cytosol, while peptides generated in the endocytic vesicles after internalisation are bound to MHC class II (MHC-II). Cellular membranes separate these two cellular environments - intracellular and extracellular. Each T cell can finally recognise only ten to hundreds copies of a unique sequence of a single peptide among thousands of other peptides presented on the very same cell because MHC molecule in one cell can bind quite a large range of peptides.

Presentation of Intracellular Antigens: Class I

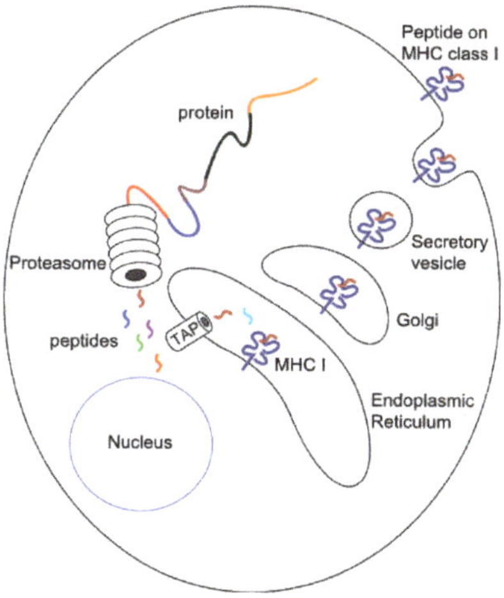

Antigen processing and presentation in MHC-I pathway

Cytotoxic T cells (also known as T_c, killer T cell, or cytotoxic T-lymphocyte (CTL)) express CD8 coreceptor are a population of T cells that are specialised for inducing programmed cell death of other cells. Cytotoxic T cells regularly patrol all body cells to maintain the organismal homeostasis. Whenever they encounter signs of disease, caused for example by the presence of viruses or intracellular bacteria or a transformed tumor cell, they initiate processes to destroy the potentially harmful cell. All nucleated cells in the body (along with platelets) display class I major histocompatibility complex (MHC-I molecules). Antigens generated endogenously within these cells are bound to MHC-I molecules and presented on the cell surface. This antigen presentation pathway enables the immune system to detect transformed or infected cells displaying peptides from modified-self (mutated) or foreign proteins.

In the presentation process, these proteins are mainly degraded into small peptides by cytosolic proteases in the proteasome, but there are also other cytoplasmic proteolytic pathways. Then, peptides are distributed to the endoplasmic reticulum via the action of heat shok proteins and the transporter associated with antigen processing (TAP) which translocates the cytosolic peptides into the ER lumen in an ATP-dependent transport mechanism. There are several ER chaperones involved in MHC-I assembly, such as calnexin, clareticulin and tapasin. Peptides are loaded to MHC-I peptide binding groove between two alpha helices at the bottom of the α1 and α2 domains of the MHC class I molecule. After releasing from tapasin, peptide-MHC-I complexes (pMHC-I) exit the ER and are transported to the cell surface by exocytic vesicles.

Naïve anti-viral T cells (CD8+) cannot directly eliminate transformed or infected cells. They have to be activated by the pMHC-I complexes of antigen-presenting cells (APCs). Here, antigen can be presented directly (as described above) or indirectly (cross-presentation) from virus-infected and non-infected cells. After the interaction between pMHC-I and TCR, in presence of costimulatory signals and/or cytokines,T cells are activated, migrate to the peripheral tissues and kill the target cells (infected or damaged cells) by inducing cytotoxicity.

Cross-presentation is a special case in which MHC-I molecules are able to present extracellular antigens, usually displayed only by MHC-II molecules. This ability appears in several APCs, mainly plasmacytoid dendritic cells in tissues that stimulate CD8+ T cells directly. This process is essential when APCs are not directly infected, triggering local antiviral and anti-tumor immune responses immediately without trafficking the APCs in the local lymph nodes.

Presentation of Extracellular Antigens: Class II

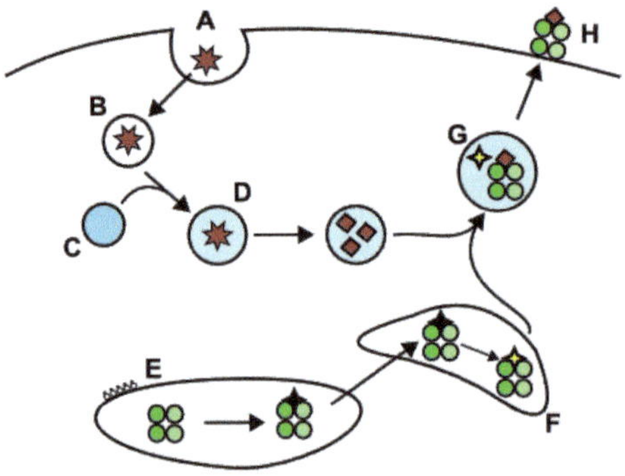

MHC II antigen processing pathway A Foreign protein; B Endosome; C Lysosome; D Late endosome/ Endolysosome; E ER; F Golgi apparatus; G CLIP for antigen exchange; H Antigen presentation at plasma membrane

Antigens from the extracellular space and sometimes also endogenous ones, are enclosed into endocytic vesicles and presented on the cell surface by MHC-II molecules to the helper T cells expressing CD4 molecule. Only APCs do express the class II of MHC molecules on the surface in large quantity, such as dendritic cells, B cells or macrophages, so expression of MHC-II molecules is more cell-specific than MHC-I.

APCs usually internalise exogenous antigens by endocytosis, but also by pinocytosis, macroautophagy, endosomal microautophagy or chaperone-mediated autophagy. In the first case, after internalisation, the antigens are enclosed in vesicles called endosomes. There are three compartements involved in this antigen presentation pathway: early endosomes, late endosomes or endolysosomes and lysosomes, where antigens are hydrolized by lysosome-associated enzymes (acid-dependent hydrolases, glycosidases, proteases, lipases). This process is favored by gradual reduction of the pH. The main proteases in endosomes are cathepsins and the result is the degradation of the antigens into oligopeptides.

MHC-II molecules are transported from the ER to the MHC class II loading compartment together with the protein Invariant chain (Ii, CD74). A non classical MHC-II molecule (HLA-DO and HLA-DM) catalyses the exchange of part of the CD74 (CLIP peptide) with the peptide antigen. Peptide-MHC-II complexes (pMHC-II) are transported to the plasma membrane and the processed antigen is presented to the helper T cells in the lymph nodes.

APCs undergo a process of maturation while migrating, via chemotactic signals, to lymphoid tissues, in which they lose the phagocytic capacity and develop an increased ability to communicate with T-cells by antigen-presentation. As well as in CD8+ cytotoxic T cells, APCs need pMHC-II and additional costimulatory signals to fully activate naive T helper cells.

Alternative pathway of endogenous antigen processing and presentation over MHC-II molecules exists in medulary thymic epithelial cells (mTEC) via the process of autophagy. It is important for the process of central tolerance of T cells in particular the negative selection of autoreactive clones. Random gene expression of the whole genome is achieved via the action of AIRE and a self-digestion of the expressed molecules presented on both MHC-I and MHC-II molecules.

Presentation of Native Intact Antigens to B Cells

B-cell receptors on the surface of B cells bind to intact native and undigested antigens of structural nature, rather than to a linear sequence of a peptide which has been digested into small fragments and presented by MHC molecules. Large complexes of intact antigen are presented in lymph nodes to B cells by follicular dendritic cells in the form of immune complexes. Some APCs expressing comparatively lower levels of lysosomal enzymes are thus less likely to digest the antigen they have captured before presenting it to B cells.

Different Stages of Adaptive Immune Response

Steps of adaptive immune response follow a cascade orchestrated by the antibodies and the cells of the adaptive immune system.

Step 1 Capture and display of antigens

↓

Step 2 Recognition of antigen by lymphocytes

↓

Step 3 Activation of T lymphocytes

↓

Step 4 Activation of B lymphocytes

↓

Step 5 Production of memory cells

Capture and Display of Antigens

Dendritic cells present in the epithelial body surfaces and connective tissues are the major antigen presenting cells. They display the antigens to the CD4+ T cells to activate the antibody mediated (humoral) immune response and CD8+ T cells to activate cell mediated immune response. The antigen presenting cells contain a specialized structure over their surface called the MHC molecules that helps in the display of antigenic peptides to the cells of immune system. Pathogens entering into lymph nodes and spleen are displayed by the antigen presenting cells to the B and T lymphocytes.

Recognition of Antigen by Lymphocytes

Lymphocyte specific for an antigen is activated upon encountering with antigen presenting cells loaded with an antigenic peptide. The concept of activation of lymphocyte is called clonal selection theory. The theory was put forth first by Neils Jerne and explained further by Burnet. This theory says that antigen specific clones of lymphocytes exist even before the exposure of antigens and a large number of clones are generated during lymphocytic maturation to diversify the recognition of microbial antigens.

Activation of T Lymphocytes

Activated T helper cells proliferate and differentiate into effector cells with the help of cytokines. Interleukin-2, secreted by T-helper cells modulate the clonal expansion of activated T lymphocytes. The effector cells help in killing the pathogen by phagocytosis.

Activated cytotoxic T cells kill the intracellular pathogens in the cytoplasm of infected cells. Alternatively, cytotoxic T cells eliminate the infection by phagocytosis of the infected cells.

Activation of B Lymphocytes

B cells are activated with the help of CD4+ T lymphocyte and differentiated into antibody secreting plasma cells. Usually lipids and carbohydrate antigens stimulate the production of IgM class of antibody while protein antigens can induce IgG, IgA, IgE type of immunoglobulins. The production of different form of antibodies requires class switching of the surface immunoglobulin present over the B cells. Antibodies bind and prevent the pathogens, thus "neutralizing" the pathogens and block their ability to infect host cells. IgA antibodies specifically act on the mucosal surface of the gastrointestinal and respiratory tract and neutralize the invading pathogens. IgG antibodies coat pathogens and target them for phagocytosis while IgM can activate the complement pathway.

Production of Memory Cells

Initial activation of T lymphocyte produces the long-lived memory cells that survive for many days following infection. Memory cells respond much faster than the naïve lymphocytes. Generations of long lasting memory cells are the major target for vaccine design against microbial pathogens.

Immune Network Theory

The immune network theory is a theory of how the adaptive immune system works, that has been developed since 1974 mainly by Niels Jerne and Geoffrey W. Hoffmann. The theory states that the immune system is an interacting network of lymphocytes and molecules that have variable (V) regions. These V regions bind not only to things that are foreign to the vertebrate, but also to other V regions within the system. The immune system is therefore seen as a network, with the components connected to each other by V-V interactions.

It has been suggested that the phenomena that the theory describes in terms of networks are also explained by clonal selection theory.

The scope of the symmetrical network theory developed by Hoffmann includes the phenomena of low dose and high dose tolerance, first reported for a single antigen by Avrion Mitchison, and confirmed by Geoffrey Shellam and Sir Gustav Nossal, the helper and suppressor roles of T cells, the role of non-specific accessory cells in immune responses, and the very important phenomenon called I-J. Jerne was awarded the Nobel Prize for Medicine or Physiology in 1984 partly for his work towards the clonal selection theory, as well as his proposal of the immune network concept.

Immune network theory has also inspired a subfield of optimization algorithms similar to artificial neural networks, and unrelated to biological immunology.

The Symmetrical Immune Network Theory

Heinz Kohler was involved in early idiotypic network research and was the first to suggest that idiotypic network interactions are symmetrical. developed a detailed immune network theory based on symmetrical stimulatory, inhibitory and killing interactions. It offers a framework for understanding a large number of immunological phenomena based on a small number of postulates. The theory involves roles for B cells that make antibodies, T cells that regulate the production of antibodies by B cells, and non-specific accessory cells (A cells).

Antibodies called IgG have two V regions and a molecular weight of 150,000. A central role in the theory is played by specific T cell factors, which have a molecular weight of approximately 50,000, and are postulated in the theory to have only one V region. Hoffmann has proposed that for brevity specific T cell factors should be called tabs. Tabs are able to exert a powerful suppressive effect on the production of IgG antibodies in response to foreign substances (antigens), as was demonstrated rigorously by Takemori and Tada. In the symmetrical network theory tabs are able to block V regions and also to have a stimulatory role when bound to a tab receptor on A cells. Symmetrical stimulatory interactions follow from the postulate that activation of B cells, T cells and A cells involves cross-linking of receptors.

The symmetrical network theory has been developed with the assistance of mathematical modeling. In order to exhibit immune memory to any combination of a large number of different pathogens, the system has a large number of stable steady states. The system is also able to switch between steady states as has been observed experimentally. For example, low or high doses of an antigen can cause the system to switch to a suppressed state for the antigen, while intermediate doses can cause the induction of immunity.

Resolution of the I-J Paradox

The theory accounts for the ability of T cells to have regulatory roles in both helping and suppressing immune responses. In 1976 two groups independently reported a phenomenon in mice called I-J. From the perspective of the symmetrical network theory, I-J is one of the most important phenomena in immunology, while for many immunologists who are not familiar with the details of the theory, I-J "does not exist". This is because I-J seemed to map to within the Major Histocompatibility Complex, and no gene could be found at the site where I-J had been mapped in numerous experiments. This became known as the "I-J paradox". This paradox resulted in suppressor T cells and tabs, which both express I-J determinants, falling out of favour, together with the symmetrical network theory, that is based on the existence of tabs. In the meantime however, it has been shown that the I-J paradox can be resolved in the context of the symmetrical network theory.

The resolution of the I-J paradox involves a process of mutual selection (or "co-selection") of suppressor T cells and helper T cells, meaning that (a) those suppressor T cells are selected that have V regions with complementarity to as many helper T cells as possible, and (b) helper T cells are selected not only on the basis of their V regions having some affinity for MHC class II, but also on the basis of the V regions having some affinity for the selected suppressor T cell V regions. The helper T cells and suppressor T cells that are co-selected are then a mutually stabilizing construct, and for a given mouse genome, more than one such mutually stabilizing set can exist. This resolution of the I-J paradox leads to some testable predictions.

Relevance for Understanding HIV Pathogenesis

An immune network model for HIV pathogenesis was published in 1994 postulating that HIV-specific T cells are preferentially infected (Hoffmann, 1994, op cit.). The publication of this paper was followed in 2002 with the publication of a paper entitled "HIV preferentially infects HIV specific CD4+ T cells."

Under the immune network theory, the main cause for progression to AIDS after HIV infection is not the direct killing of infected T helper cells by the virus. Following an infection with HIV that manages to establish itself, there is a complex interaction between the HIV virus, the T helper cells that it infects, and T suppressor cells. These three quasispecies apply selective pressure on one another and co-evolve in such a way that the viral epitopes eventually come to mimick the V regions of the main population of T suppressor cells. Once this happens, anti-HIV antibodies can bind to and kill most of the host's T suppressor cell population. This results in the dysregulation of the immune system, and eventually to other further anti-self reactions, including against the T helper cell population. At that point, the adaptive immune system is completely compromised and AIDS ensues. Hence in this model, the onset of AIDS is primarily an auto-immune reaction triggered by the cross-reaction of anti-HIV antibodies with T suppressor cells. Once this induced auto-immunity sets in, removing the HIV virus itself (for instance via HAART) would not be sufficient to restore proper immune function. The co-evolution of the quasispecies mentioned above will take a variable time depending on the initial conditions at the time of infection (i.e. the epitopes of the first infection and the steady state of the host's immune cell population), which would explain why there is a variable period, which differs greatly between individual patients, between HIV infection and the onset of AIDS. It also suggests that conventional vaccines are unlikely to be successful, since they would not prevent the auto-immune reaction. In fact such vaccines may do more harm in certain cases, since if the original infection comes from a source with a "mature" infection, those virions will have a high affinity for anti-HIV T helper cells, and so increasing the anti-HIV population via vaccination only serves to provide the virus with more easy targets.

HIV Vaccine Based on Immune Network Theory

An HIV vaccine concept based on immune network theory has been described. The vaccine concept was based on a network theory resolution of the Oudin-Cazenave paradox. This is a phenomenon that makes no sense in the context of clonal selection, without taking idiotypic network interactions into account. The vaccine concept comprised complexes of an anti-anti-HIV antibody and an HIV antigen, and was designed to induce the production of broadly neutralizing anti-HIV antibodies. A suitable anti-anti-HIV antibody envisaged for use in this vaccine is the monoclonal antibody 1F7, which was discovered by Sybille Muller and Heinz Kohler and their colleagues. This monoclonal antibody binds to all of six well characterized broadly neutralizing anti-HIV antibodies.

MHC Restriction of V-V Interactions in Serum IgG

IgG from mice with a given set of MHC genes binds rapidly and specifically in an ELISA assay to IgG from mice with the same MHC, but not to IgG from mice with different MHC genes. An idiotypic network model based on co-selection provides an explanation for this phenomenon. In the model IgG molecules are selected to have both anti-anti-(self MHC class II) and anti-anti-anti-(self MHC class II) specificity, and therefore have MHC-restricted self-binding.

References

- Belikov, Aleksey V.; Schraven, Burkhart; Simeoni, Luca (1 January 2015). "T cells and reactive oxygen species". Journal of Biomedical Science. 22: 85. ISSN 1423-0127. PMID 26471060. doi:10.1186/s12929-015-0194-3. Retrieved 29 April 2017
- Alberts, B.; Johnson, A.; Lewis, J.; Raff, M.; Roberts, K.; Walters, P. (2002). Molecular Biology of the Cell (4th ed.). New York and London: Garland Science. ISBN 0-8153-3218-1
- Williams TN, Mwangi TW, Roberts DJ, Alexander ND, Weatherall DJ, Wambua S, Kortok M, Snow RW, Marsh K (2005). "An Immune Basis for Malaria Protection by the Sickle Cell Trait". PLoS Med. 2 (5): e128. PMC 1140945 . PMID 15916466. doi:10.1371/journal.pmed.0020128
- Janeway, C.A.; Travers, P.; Walport, M.; Shlomchik, M.J. (2001). Immunobiology (5th ed.). New York and London: Garland Science. ISBN 0-8153-4101-6
- "The melting pot of the MHC II peptidome". Current Opinion in Immunology. 40: 70–77. doi:10.1016/j.coi.2016.03.004. Retrieved 2017-01-04
- Willinger T, Freeman T, Hasegawa H, McMichael AJ, Callan MF (2005). "Molecular signatures distinguish human central memory from effector memory CD8 T cell subsets.". Journal of Immunology. 175 (9): 5895–903. PMID 16237082. doi:10.4049/jimmunol.175.9.5895
- Janeway, C.A.; Travers, P.; Walport, M.; Shlomchik, M.J. (2005). Immunobiology. (6th ed.). Garland Science. ISBN 0-443-07310-4
- Batista, Facundo D.; Harwood, Naomi E. (January 2009). "The who, how and where of antigen presentation to B cells". Nature Reviews Immunology. Macmillan Publishers Limited. 9: 15–27. doi:10.1038/nri2454. Retrieved 25 May 2016
- Murphy, Kenneth (2012). Janeway's Immunobiology 8th Edition. New York, NY: Garland Science. ISBN 9780815342434
- "The melting pot of the MHC II peptidome". Current Opinion in Immunology. 40: 70–77. doi:10.1016/j.coi.2016.03.004. Retrieved 2017-01-04
- Janeway, Charles; Travers, Paul; Walport, Mark; Shlomchik, Mark (2001). Immunobiology (5th ed.). New York and London: Garland Science. ISBN 0-8153-4101-6
- Overgaard, Nana H.; Jung, Ji-Won; Steptoe, Raymond J.; Wells, James W. (1 January 2015). "CD4+/CD8+ double-positive T cells: more than just a developmental stage?". Journal of Leukocyte Biology. 97 (1): 31–38. ISSN 1938-3673. PMID 25360000. doi:10.1189/jlb.1RU0814-382
- Abbas, A. K.; Lichtman, A. H. (2003). Cellular and Molecular Immunology (5th ed.). Saunders, Philadelphia. ISBN 0-7216-0008-5

4

A Brief Introduction to Cytokine

Cytokines are important for cell signaling. They are proteins that regulate the immune response. A few features of cytokines are that they are secreted in large number by the immune system; they are highly toxic if taken in huge amounts; and they show redundancy. The chapter on cytokines offers an insightful focus, keeping in mind the complex subject matter.

Cytokine

Cytokines are a broad and loose category of small proteins (~5–20 kDa) that are important in cell signaling. Their release has an effect on the behavior of cells around them. It can be said that cytokines are involved in autocrine signalling, paracrine signalling and endocrine signalling as immunomodulating agents. Their definite distinction from hormones is still part of ongoing research. Cytokines include chemokines, interferons, interleukins, lymphokines, and tumour necrosis factors but generally not hormones or growth factors (despite some overlap in the terminology). Cytokines are produced by a broad range of cells, including immune cells like macrophages, B lymphocytes, T lymphocytes and mast cells, as well as endothelial cells, fibroblasts, and various stromal cells; a given cytokine may be produced by more than one type of cell.

They act through receptors, and are especially important in the immune system; cytokines modulate the balance between humoral and cell-based immune responses, and they regulate the maturation, growth, and responsiveness of particular cell populations. Some cytokines enhance or inhibit the action of other cytokines in complex ways.

They are different from hormones, which are also important cell signaling molecules, in that hormones circulate in less variable concentrations and hormones tend to be made by specific kinds of cells.

They are important in health and disease, specifically in host responses to infection, immune responses, inflammation, trauma, sepsis, cancer, and reproduction.

Discovery of Cytokines

Interferon-alpha, an interferon type I, was identified in 1957 as a protein that interfered with viral replication. The activity of interferon-gamma (the sole member of the interferon type II class) was described in 1965; this was the first identified lymphocyte-derived mediator. Macrophage migration inhibitory factor (MIF) was identified simultaneously in 1966 by John David and Barry Bloom.

In 1969 Dudley Dumonde proposed the term "lymphokine" to describe proteins secreted from lymphocytes and later, proteins derived from macrophages and monocytes in culture were called "monokines". As scientists learned more, it was understood that these proteins and others were part of a broader class of proteins involved in self-defense, and should be called "cytokines".

Difference from Hormones

Classic hormones circulate in nanomolar (10^{-9} M) concentrations that usually vary by less than one order of magnitude. In contrast, some cytokines (such as IL-6) circulate in picomolar (10^{-12} M) concentrations that can increase up to 1,000-fold during trauma or infection. The widespread distribution of cellular sources for cytokines may be a feature that differentiates them from hormones. Virtually all nucleated cells, but especially endo/epithelial cells and resident macrophages (many near the interface with the external environment) are potent producers of IL-1, IL-6, and TNF-α. In contrast, classic hormones, such as insulin, are secreted from discrete glands (e.g., the pancreas). As of 2008, the current terminology refers to cytokines as immunomodulating agents. However, more research is needed in this area of defining cytokines and hormones.

Part of the difficulty with distinguishing cytokines from hormones is that some of the immunomodulating effects of cytokines are systemic rather than local. For instance, to use hormone terminology, the action of cytokines may be autocrine or paracrine in chemotaxis or chemokinesis and endocrine as a pyrogen. Further, as molecules, cytokines are not limited to their immunomodulatory role.

Nomenclature

Cytokines have been classed as lymphokines, interleukins, and chemokines, based on their presumed function, cell of secretion, or target of action. Because cytokines are characterised by considerable redundancy and pleiotropism, such distinctions, allowing for exceptions, are obsolete.

- The term *interleukin* was initially used by researchers for those cytokines whose presumed targets are principally leukocytes. It is now used largely for designation of newer cytokine molecules and bears little relation to their presumed function. The vast majority of these are produced by T-helper cells.
- *Lymphokines*, produced by lymphocytes
- *Monokines*, produced exclusively by monocytes
- *Interferons*, involved in antiviral responses

- *Colony stimulating factors*, support the growth of cells in semisolid media
- *Chemokines* mediate chemoattraction (chemotaxis) between cells.

Classification

Structural

Structural homogeneity has been able to partially distinguish between cytokines that do not demonstrate a considerable degree of redundancy so that they can be classified into four types:

- The four-α-helix bundle family: member cytokines have three-dimensional structures with four bundles of α-helices. This family, in turn, is divided into three sub-families:
    1. the IL-2 subfamily
    2. the interferon (IFN) subfamily
    3. the IL-10 subfamily.
        - The first of these three, the IL-2 subfamily, is the largest. It contains several non-immunological cytokines including erythropoietin (EPO) and thrombopoietin (TPO). Furthermore, four-α-helix bundle cytokines can be grouped into *long-chain* and *short-chain* cytokines.
- the IL-1 family, which primarily includes IL-1 and IL-18
- the IL-17 family, which has yet to be completely characterized, though member cytokines have a specific effect in promoting proliferation of T-cells that cause cytotoxic effects.
- the cysteine-knot cytokines include members of the transforming-growth-factor-beta superfamily, including TGF-β1, TGF-β2 and TGF-β3.

Functional

A classification that proves more useful in clinical and experimental practice outside of structural biology divides immunological cytokines into those that enhance cellular immune responses, type 1 (TNFα, IFN-γ, etc.), and type 2 (TGF-β, IL-4, IL-10, IL-13, etc.), which favor antibody responses.

A key focus of interest has been that cytokines in one of these two sub-sets tend to inhibit the effects of those in the other. Dysregulation of this tendency is under intensive study for its possible role in the pathogenesis of autoimmune disorders.

Several inflammatory cytokines are induced by oxidative stress. The fact that cytokines themselves trigger the release of other cytokines and also lead to increased oxidative stress makes them important in chronic inflammation, as well as other immunoresponses, such as fever and acute phase proteins of the liver (IL-1,6,12, IFN-a).

Cytokines also play a role in anti-inflammatory pathways and are a possible therapeutic treatment for pathological pain from inflammation or peripheral nerve injury. There are both pro-inflammatory and anti-inflammatory cytokines that regulate this pathway.

Receptors

In recent years, the cytokine receptors have come to demand the attention of more investigators than cytokines themselves, partly because of their remarkable characteristics, and partly because a deficiency of cytokine receptors has now been directly linked to certain debilitating immunodeficiency states. In this regard, and also because the redundancy and pleomorphism of cytokines are, in fact, a consequence of their homologous receptors, many authorities think that a classification of cytokine receptors would be more clinically and experimentally useful.

A classification of cytokine receptors based on their three-dimensional structure has, therefore, been attempted. Such a classification, though seemingly cumbersome, provides several unique perspectives for attractive pharmacotherapeutic targets.

- Immunoglobulin (Ig) superfamily, which are ubiquitously present throughout several cells and tissues of the vertebrate body, and share structural homology with immunoglobulins (antibodies), cell adhesion molecules, and even some cytokines. Examples: IL-1 receptor types.
- Hemopoietic Growth Factor (type 1) family, whose members have certain conserved motifs in their extracellular amino-acid domain. The IL-2 receptor belongs to this chain, whose γ-chain (common to several other cytokines) deficiency is directly responsible for the x-linked form of Severe Combined Immunodeficiency (X-SCID).
- Interferon (type 2) family, whose members are receptors for IFN β and γ.
- Tumor necrosis factors (TNF) (type 3) family, whose members share a cysteine-rich common extracellular binding domain, and includes several other non-cytokine ligands like CD40, CD27 and CD30, besides the ligands on which the family is named (TNF).
- Seven transmembrane helix family, the ubiquitous receptor type of the animal kingdom. All G protein-coupled receptors (for hormones and neurotransmitters) belong to this family. Chemokine receptors, two of which act as binding proteins for HIV (CD4 and CCR5), also belong to this family.
- Interleukin-17 receptor (IL-17R) family, which shows little homology with any other cytokine receptor family. Structural motifs conserved between members of this family include: an extracellular fibronectin III-like domain, a trans-

membrane domain and a cytoplasmic SERIF domain. The known members of this family are as follows: IL-17RA, IL-17RB, IL-17RC, IL17RD and IL-17RE.

Cellular Effects

Each cytokine has a matching cell-surface receptor. Subsequent cascades of intracellular signalling then alter cell functions. This may include the upregulation and/or downregulation of several genes and their transcription factors, resulting in the production of other cytokines, an increase in the number of surface receptors for other molecules, or the suppression of their own effect by feedback inhibition.

The effect of a particular cytokine on a given cell depends on the cytokine, its extracellular abundance, the presence and abundance of the complementary receptor on the cell surface, and downstream signals activated by receptor binding; these last two factors can vary by cell type. Cytokines are characterized by considerable "redundancy", in that many cytokines appear to share similar functions.

It seems to be a paradox that cytokines binding to antibodies have a stronger immune effect than the cytokine alone. This may lead to lower therapeutic doses.

Said et al. showed that inflammatory cytokines cause an IL-10-dependent inhibition of T-cell expansion and function by up-regulating PD-1 levels on monocytes which leads to IL-10 production by monocytes after binding of PD-1 by PD-L.

Adverse reactions to cytokines are characterized by local inflammation and/or ulceration at the injection sites. Occasionally such reactions are seen with more widespread papular eruptions.

Roles of Endogenous Cytokines in Health and Disease

Cytokines are often involved in several developmental processes during embryogenesis.

Cytokines are crucial for fighting off infections and in other immune responses. However, they can become dysregulated and pathological in inflammation, trauma, and sepsis.

Adverse effects of cytokines have been linked to many disease states and conditions ranging from schizophrenia, major depression and Alzheimer's disease to cancer. Normal tissue integrity is preserved by feedback interactions between diverse cell types mediated by adhesion molecules and secreted cytokines; disruption of normal feedback mechanisms in cancer threatens tissue integrity. Over-secretion of cytokines can trigger a dangerous syndrome known as a cytokine storm; this may have been the cause of severe adverse events during a clinical trial of TGN1412. Cytokine storms are suspected to be the main cause of death in the 1918 "Spanish Flu" pandemic. Deaths were weighted more heavily towards people with healthy immune systems, due to its ability to produce stronger immune responses, likely increasing cytokine levels. Another important example of cytokine storm is seen in acute pancreatitis. Cytokines are integral and implicated in all angles of the cascade resulting in the systemic inflammatory response syndrome and multi organ failure associated with this intra-abdominal catastrophe.

Medical use as Drugs

Some cytokines have been developed into protein therapeutics using recombinant DNA technology. Recombinant cytokines being used as drugs as of 2014 include:

- Bone morphogenetic protein (BMP), used to treat bone-related conditions
- Erythropoietin (EPO), used to treat anemia
- Granulocyte colony-stimulating factor (G-CSF), used to treat neutropenia in cancer patients
- Granulocyte macrophage colony-stimulating factor (GM-CSF), used to treat neutropenia and fungal infections in cancer patients
- Interferon alfa, used to treat hepatitis C and multiple scelerosis
- Interferon beta, used to treat multiple scelerosis
- Interleukin 2 (IL-2), used to treat cancer.
- Interleukin 11 (IL-11), used to treat thrombocytopenia in cancer patients.
- Interferon gamma is used to treat chronic granulomatous disease and osteopetrosis

Research into Diagnostic Use of Measured Levels

Plasma levels of various cytokines may give information on the presence, or even predictive value of inflammatory processes involved in autoimmune diseases such as rheumatoid arthritis, as well as immunomodulatory effects of foods or drugs. In addition, elevated levels of IL-7, an important cytokine involved in T cell homeostasis, have been detected in the plasma of HIV-infected patients.

Features of Cytokines

1) Cytokines show redundancy i.e. different cytokines may have similar function, e.g. IL-1 and IL-6 both induce fever by acting on brain.

2) They are secreted in multiple numbers, e.g. macrophages secrete more than five interleukins and tumor necrosis factor.

3) Cytokines produce their effect on many cell types i.e. they are pleiotropic.

4) Cytokines need extreme regulation and are toxic in high doses.

Cytokine Nomenclature

Most of the cytokines are named according to the Interleukin nomenclature subcommittee of the international union of immunological societies. Although the definition of cytokines is quite broad, but together they can be classified as lymphokines, interleukins, interferons , chemokines etc. depending on their function, cell of secretion, or target of action. The name interleukin was coined initially for those cytokines that mediate signaling between lymphocytes and leukocytes. In other words leukocytes were thought to be the principal target for interleukins but now this definition is no longer in function and the name interleukin is given to any new cytokine discovered routinely. Cytokines are produced mainly in response to viral infection or in response to immune attack. Interferons are the cytokines that interfere with viral RNA and protein synthesis to prevent viral replication.

Types of interferon – Interferons are mainly divided into two types.

Type I Interferons --- Interferon-α (IFN- α) and interferon-β (IFN-β).

Type II interferon --- Interferon-γ

Tumor necrosis factors (TNFs) can kill tumor cells and colony stimulating factors assist in regulation of stem cell activities. Chemokines play role in leukocyte recruitment and circulation.

Table: Different cytokines and their examples:

Cytokine types	Examples
Lymphokines	MAF (Macrophage activating factor)
Interleukins	IL-7, IL-13, IL1-7
Interferons	IFN-α, IFN –β, IFN-γ, IFN-ω, IFN -
Tumor necrosis factors	TNF- α (Cachectin), TNF – β (lymphotoxin)
Colony stimulating factors	GSF (Granulocyte colony stimulating factor)
Polypeptide growth factors	EGF (Epidermal growth factor)
α-Chemokines	PF-4 (Platelet factor 4)
β-Chemokines	MCP-1 (Monocyte chemoattractant protein 1)
Transforming growth factors	TGF- α, TGF - β
Stress proteins	Heat shock proteins
RANTES	

Lymphokine

Lymphokines are a subset of cytokines that are produced by a type of immune cell known as a lymphocyte. They are protein mediators typically produced by T cells to direct the immune system response by signaling between its cells. Lymphokines have many roles, including the attraction of other immune cells, including macrophages and other lymphocytes, to an infected site and their subsequent activation to prepare them to mount an immune response. Circulating lymphocytes can detect a very small concentration of lymphokine and then move up the concentration gradient towards where the immune response is required. Lymphokines aid B cells to produce antibodies.

Important lymphokines secreted by the T helper cell include:

- Interleukin 2
- Interleukin 3
- Interleukin 4
- Interleukin 5
- Interleukin 6
- Granulocyte-macrophage colony-stimulating factor
- Interferon-gamma

Chemokine

Chemokines (movement) are a family of small cytokines, or signaling proteins secreted by cells. Their name is derived from their ability to induce directed chemotaxis in nearby responsive cells; they are chemotactic cytokines.

Cytokine proteins are classified as chemokines according to behavior and structural characteristics. In addition to being known for mediating chemotaxis, chemokines are all approximately 8-10 kilodaltons in mass and have four cysteine residues in conserved locations that are key to forming their 3-dimensional shape.

These proteins have historically been known under several other names including the *SIS family of cytokines, SIG family of cytokines, SCY family of cytokines, Platelet factor-4 superfamily* or *intercrines*. Some chemokines are considered pro-inflammatory and can be induced during an immune response to recruit cells of the immune system to a site of infection, while others are considered homeostatic and are involved in controlling the migration of cells during normal processes of tissue maintenance or development. Chemokines are found in all vertebrates, some viruses and some bacteria, but none have been described for other invertebrates.

Chemokines have been classified into four main subfamilies: CXC, CC, CX3C and XC.

All of these proteins exert their biological effects by interacting with G protein-linked transmembrane receptors called chemokine receptors, that are selectively found on the surfaces of their target cells.

Function

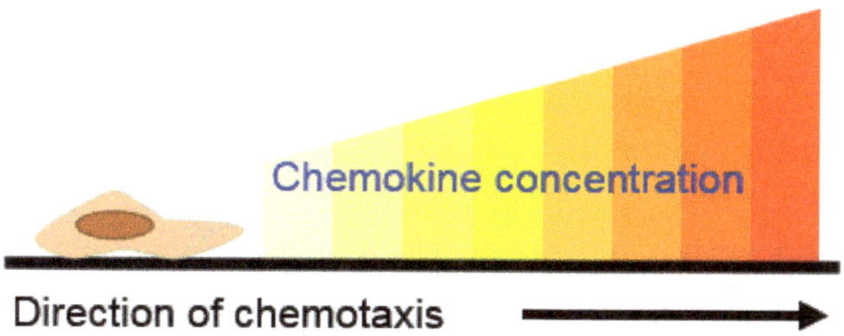

Chemokines released by infected or damaged cells form a concentration gradient. Attracted cells move through the gradient towards the higher concentration of chemokine.

The major role of chemokines is to act as a chemoattractant to guide the migration of cells. Cells that are attracted by chemokines follow a signal of increasing chemokine concentration towards the source of the chemokine. Some chemokines control cells of the immune system during processes of immune surveillance, such as directing lymphocytes to the lymph nodes so they can screen for invasion of pathogens by interacting with antigen-presenting cells residing in these tissues. These are known as homeostatic chemokines and are produced and secreted without any need to stimulate their source cell(s). Some chemokines have roles in development; they promote angiogenesis (the growth of new blood vessels), or guide cells to tissues that provide specific signals critical for cellular maturation. Other chemokines are inflammatory and are released from a wide variety of cells in response to bacterial infection, viruses and agents that cause physical damage such as silica or the urate crystals that occur in gout. Their release is often stimulated by pro-inflammatory cytokines such as interleukin 1. Inflammatory chemokines function mainly as chemoattractants for leukocytes, recruiting monocytes, neutrophils and other effector cells from the blood to sites of infection or tissue damage. Certain inflammatory chemokines activate cells to initiate an immune response or promote wound healing. They are released by many different cell types and serve to guide cells of both innate immune system and adaptive immune system.

Types by function

Chemokines are functionally divided into two groups:

- Homeostatic: are constitutively produced in certain tissues and are responsible for basal leukocyte migration. These include: CCL14, CCL19, CCL20, CCL21, CCL25, CCL27, CXCL12 and CXCL13. This classification is not strict; for example, CCL20 can act also as pro-inflammatory chemokine.
- Inflammatory: these are formed under pathological conditions (on pro-inflam-

matory stimuli, such as IL-1, TNF-alpha, LPS, or viruses) and actively participate in the inflammatory response attracting immune cells to the site of inflammation. Examples are: CXCL-8, CCL2, CCL3, CCL4, CCL5, CCL11, CXCL10.

Homing

The main function of chemokines is to manage the migration of leukocytes (homing) in the respective anatomical locations in inflammatory and homeostatic processes.

Basal: homeostatic chemokines are basal produced in the thymus and lymphoid tissues. Their homeostatic function in homing is best exemplified by the chemokines CCL19 and CCL21 (expressed within lymph nodes and on lymphatic endothelial cells) and their receptor CCR7 (expressed on cells destined for homing in cells to these organs). Using these ligands is possible routing antigen-presenting cells (APC) to lymph nodes during the adaptive immune response. Among other homeostatic chemokine receptors include: CCR9, CCR10, and CXCR5, which are important as part of the cell addresses for tissue-specific homing of leukocytes. CCR9 supports the migration of leukocytes into the intestine, CCR10 to the skin and CXCR5 supports the migration of B-cell to follicles of lymph nodes. As well CXCL12 (SDF-1) constitutively produced in the bone marrow promotes proliferation of progenitor B cells in the bone marrow microenvironment.

Inflammatory: inflammatory chemokines are produced in high concentrations during infection or injury and determine the migration of inflammatory leukocytes into the damaged area. Typical inflammatory chemokines include: CCL2, CCL3 and CCL5, CXCL1, CXCL2 and CXCL8. A typical example is CXCL-8, which chemoatractants for neutrophils. In contrast to the homeostatic chemokine receptors, there is significantly promiscuous (redundancy) binding receptor and inflammatory chemokines. This often complicated research on receptor-specific therapeutics in this area.

Types by cell attracted

- Monocytes / macrophages: the key chemokines that attract these cells to the site of inflammation include: CCL2, CCL3, CCL5, CCL7, CCL8, CCL13, CCL17 and CCL22.
- T-lymphocytes: the four key chemokines that are involved in the recruitment of T lymphocytes to the site of inflammation are: CCL2, CCL1, CCL22 and CCL17.
- Mast cells: on their surface express several receptors for chemokines: CCR1, CCR2, CCR3, CCR4, CCR5, CXCR2, and CXCR4. Ligands of these receptors CCL2 and CCL5 play an important role in mast cell recruitment and activation in the lung.There is also evidence that CXCL8 might be inhibitory of mast cell.
- Eosinophils: the migration of eosinophils into various tissues involved several

chemokines of CC family: CCL11, CCL24, CCL26, CCL5, CCL7, CCL13, and CCL3. Chemokines CCL11 (eotaxin) and CCL5 (RANTES) acts through a specific receptor CCR3 on the surface of eosinophils, and eotaxin plays an essential role in the initial recruitment of eosinophils into the lesion.

- Neutrophils: are regulated primarily by CXC chemokines. An example CXCL8 (IL-8) is chemoattractant for neutrophils and also activating their metabolic and degranulation.

Structural Characteristics

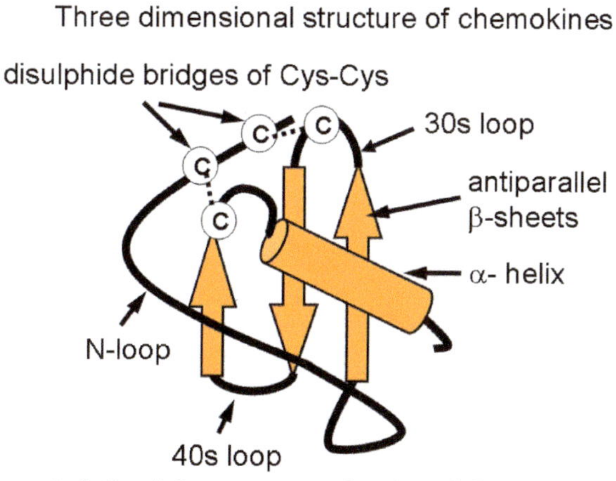

All chemokines share a typical *Greek key* structure that is stabilised by disulfide bonds between conserved cysteine residues.

Proteins are classified into the chemokine family based on their structural characteristics, not just their ability to attract cells. All chemokines are small, with a molecular mass of between 8 and 10 kDa. They are approximately 20-50% identical to each other; that is, they share gene sequence and amino acid sequence homology. They all also possess conserved amino acids that are important for creating their 3-dimensional or tertiary structure, such as (in most cases) four cysteines that interact with each other in pairs to create a Greek key shape that is a characteristic of chemokines. Intramolecular disulfide bonds typically join the first to third, and the second to fourth cysteine residues, numbered as they appear in the protein sequence of the chemokine. Typical chemokine proteins are produced as pro-peptides, beginning with a signal peptide of approximately 20 amino acids that gets cleaved from the active (mature) portion of the molecule during the process of its secretion from the cell. The first two cysteines, in a chemokine, are situated close together near the N-terminal end of the mature protein, with the third cysteine residing in the centre of the molecule and the fourth close to the C-terminal end. A loop of approximately ten amino acids follows the first two cysteines and is known as the *N-loop*. This is followed by a single-turn helix, called a 3_{10}-helix, three β-strands and a C-terminal α-helix. These helices and strands are connected by turns called *30s*, *40s* and *50s* loops; the third and fourth cysteines are located in the 30s and 50s loops.

Types by Structure

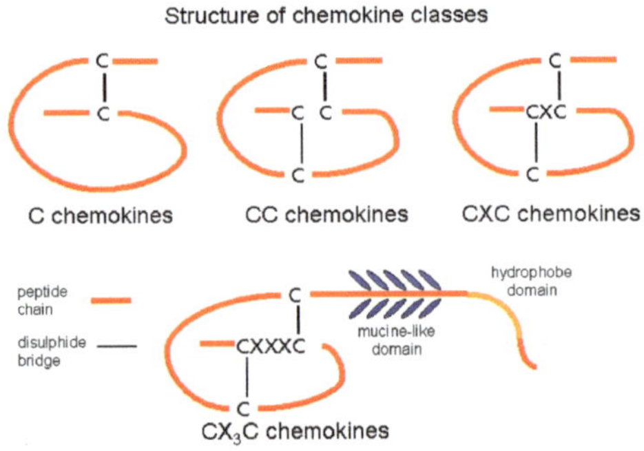

CC chemokines				
Name	**Gene**	**Other name(s)**	**Receptor**	**Uniprot**
CCL1	Scya1	I-309, TCA-3	CCR8	
CCL2	Scya2	MCP-1	CCR2	P13500
CCL3	Scya3	MIP-1a	CCR1	P10147
CCL4	Scya4	MIP-1β	CCR1, CCR5	P13236
CCL5	Scya5	RANTES	CCR5	P13501
CCL6	Scya6	C10, MRP-2	CCR1	P27784
CCL7	Scya7	MARC, MCP-3	CCR2	P80098
CCL8	Scya8	MCP-2	CCR1, CCR2B, CCR5	P80075
CCL9/CCL10	Scya9	MRP-2, CCF18, MIP-1?	CCR1	P51670
CCL11	Scya11	Eotaxin	CCR2, CCR3, CCR5	P51671
CCL12	Scya12	MCP-5		Q62401
CCL13	Scya13	MCP-4, NCC-1, Ckβ10	CCR2, CCR3, CCR5	Q99616
CCL14	Scya14	HCC-1, MCIF, Ckβ1, NCC-2, CCL	CCR1	Q16627
CCL15	Scya15	Leukotactin-1, MIP-5, HCC-2, NCC-3	CCR1, CCR3	Q16663
CCL16	Scya16	LEC, NCC-4, LMC, Ckβ12	CCR1, CCR2, CCR5, CCR8	O15467
CCL17	Scya17	TARC, dendrokine, ABCD-2	CCR4	Q92583
CCL18	Scya18	PARC, DC-CK1, AMAC-1, Ckβ7, MIP-4		P55774
CCL19	Scya19	ELC, Exodus-3, Ckβ11	CCR7	Q99731
CCL20	Scya20	LARC, Exodus-1, Ckβ4	CCR6	P78556
CCL21	Scya21	SLC, 6Ckine, Exodus-2, Ckβ9, TCA-4	CCR7	O00585
CCL22	Scya22	MDC, DC/β-CK	CCR4	O00626
CCL23	Scya23	MPIF-1, Ckβ8, MIP-3, MPIF-1	CCR1	P55773
CCL24	Scya24	Eotaxin-2, MPIF-2, Ckβ6	CCR3	O00175
CCL25	Scya25	TECK, Ckβ15	CCR9	O15444
CCL26	Scya26	Eotaxin-3, MIP-4a, IMAC, TSC-1	CCR3	Q9Y258
CCL27	Scya27	CTACK, ILC, Eskine, PESKY, skinkine	CCR10	Q9Y4X3
CCL28	Scya28	MEC	CCR3, CCR10	Q9NRJ3
CXCL1	Scyb1	Gro-a, GRO1, NAP-3, KC	CXCR2	P09341

CXC chemokines				
Name	**Gene**	**Other name(s)**	**Receptor**	**Uniprot**
CXCL2	Scyb2	Gro-β, GRO2, MIP-2a	CXCR2	P19875
CXCL3	Scyb3	Gro-?, GRO3, MIP-2β	CXCR2	P19876
CXCL4	Scyb4	PF-4	CXCR3B	P02776
CXCL5	Scyb5	ENA-78	CXCR2	P42830
CXCL6	Scyb6	GCP-2	CXCR1, CXCR2	P80162
CXCL7	Scyb7	NAP-2, CTAPIII, β-Ta, PEP		P02775
CXCL8	Scyb8	IL-8, NAP-1, MDNCF, GCP-1	CXCR1, CXCR2	P10145
CXCL9	Scyb9	MIG, CRG-10	CXCR3	Q07325
CXCL10	Scyb10	IP-10, CRG-2	CXCR3	P02778
CXCL11	Scyb11	I-TAC, β-R1, IP-9	CXCR3, CXCR7	O14625
CXCL12	Scyb12	SDF-1, PBSF	CXCR4, CXCR7	P48061
CXCL13	Scyb13	BCA-1, BLC	CXCR5	O43927
CXCL14	Scyb14	BRAK, bolekine		O95715
CXCL15	Scyb15	Lungkine, WECHE		Q9WVL7
CXCL16	Scyb16	SRPSOX	CXCR6	Q9H2A7
CXCL17	VCC-1	DMC, VCC-1		Q6UXB2
C chemokines				
Name	**Gene**	**Other name(s)**	**Receptor**	**Uniprot**
XCL1	Scyc1	Lymphotactin a, SCM-1a, ATAC	XCR1	P47992
XCL2	Scyc2	Lymphotactin β, SCM-1β	XCR1	Q9UBD3
CX3C chemokines				
Name	**Gene**	**Other name(s)**	**Receptor**	**Uniprot**
CX3CL1	Scyd1	Fractalkine, Neurotactin, ABCD-3	CX3CR1	P78423

Members of the chemokine family are divided into four groups depending on the spacing of their first two cysteine residues. Thus the nomenclature for chemokines is, e.g.: CCL1 for the ligand 1 of the CC-family of chemokines, and CCR1 for its respective receptor.

CC Chemokines

The CC chemokine (or β-chemokine) proteins have two adjacent cysteines (amino acids), near their amino terminus. There have been at least 27 distinct members of this subgroup reported for mammals, called CC chemokine ligands (CCL)-1 to -28; CCL10 is the same as CCL9. Chemokines of this subfamily usually contain four cysteines (C4-CC chemokines), but a small number of CC chemokines possess six cysteines (C6-CC chemokines). C6-CC chemokines include CCL1, CCL15, CCL21, CCL23 and CCL28. CC chemokines induce the migration of monocytes and other cell types such as NK cells and dendritic cells.

Examples of CC chemokine include monocyte chemoattractant protein-1 (MCP-1 or CCL2) which induces monocytes to leave the bloodstream and enter the surrounding tissue to become tissue macrophages.

CCL5 (or RANTES) attracts cells such as T cells, eosinophils and basophils that express the receptor CCR5.

Increased CCL11 levels in blood plasma are associated with aging (and reduced neurogenesis) in mice and humans.

CXC Chemokines

The two N-terminal cysteines of CXC chemokines (or α-chemokines) are separated by one amino acid, represented in this name with an "X". There have been 17 different CXC chemokines described in mammals, that are subdivided into two categories, those with a specific amino acid sequence (or motif) of glutamic acid-leucine-arginine (or ELR for short) immediately before the first cysteine of the CXC motif (ELR-positive), and those without an ELR motif (ELR-negative). ELR-positive CXC chemokines specifically induce the migration of neutrophils, and interact with chemokine receptors CXCR1 and CXCR2. An example of an ELR-positive CXC chemokine is interleukin-8 (IL-8), which induces neutrophils to leave the bloodstream and enter into the surrounding tissue. Other CXC chemokines that lack the ELR motif, such as CXCL13, tend to be chemoattractant for lymphocytes. CXC chemokines bind to CXC chemokine receptors, of which seven have been discovered to date, designated CXCR1-7.

C Chemokines

The third group of chemokines is known as the C chemokines (or γ chemokines), and is unlike all other chemokines in that it has only two cysteines; one N-terminal cysteine and one cysteine downstream. Two chemokines have been described for this subgroup and are called XCL1 (lymphotactin-α) and XCL2 (lymphotactin-β).

CX3C Chemokines

A fourth group has also been discovered and members have three amino acids between the two cysteines and is termed CX_3C chemokine (or d-chemokines). The only CX_3C chemokine discovered to date is called fractalkine (or CX_3CL1). It is both secreted and tethered to the surface of the cell that expresses it, thereby serving as both a chemoattractant and as an adhesion molecule.

Receptors

Chemokine receptors are G protein-coupled receptors containing 7 transmembrane domains that are found on the surface of leukocytes. Approximately 19 different chemokine receptors have been characterized to date, which are divided into four families depending on the type of chemokine they bind; CXCR that bind CXC chemokines, CCR that bind CC chemokines, CX3CR1 that binds the sole CX3C chemokine (CX3CL1), and XCR1 that binds the two XC chemokines (XCL1 and XCL2). They share many structural features; they are similar in size (with about 350 amino acids), have a short, acidic N-terminal end, seven helical transmembrane domains with three intracellular and three extracellular hydrophilic loops, and an intracellular C-terminus containing serine and threonine residues important for receptor regulation. The first two extracellular loops of chemokine receptors each has a conserved cysteine residue that allow formation of a disulfide bridge between these loops. G proteins are coupled to the C-terminal end of the chemokine receptor to allow intracellular signaling after receptor activation, while the N-terminal domain of the chemokine receptor determines ligand binding specificity.

Signal Transduction

Chemokine receptors associate with G-proteins to transmit cell signals following ligand binding. Activation of G proteins, by chemokine receptors, causes the subsequent activation of an enzyme known as phospholipase C (PLC). PLC cleaves a molecule called phosphatidylinositol (4,5)-bisphosphate (PIP2) into two second messenger molecules known as Inositol triphosphate (IP3) and diacylglycerol (DAG) that trigger intracellular signaling events; DAG activates another enzyme called protein kinase C (PKC), and IP3 triggers the release of calcium from intracellular stores. These events promote many signaling cascades (such as the MAP kinase pathway) that generate responses like chemotaxis, degranulation, release of superoxide anions and changes in the avidity of cell adhesion molecules called integrins within the cell harbouring the chemokine receptor.

Infection Control

The discovery that the β chemokines RANTES, MIP (macrophage inflammatory proteins) 1α and 1β (now known as CCL5, CCL3 and CCL4 respectively) suppress HIV-1 provided the initial connection and indicated that these molecules might control infection as part of immune responses in vivo, and that sustained delivery of such inhibitors have the capacity of long-term infection control. The association of chemokine production with antigen-induced proliferative responses, more favorable clinical status in HIV infection, as well as with an uninfected status in subjects at risk for infection suggests a positive role for these molecules in controlling the natural course of HIV infection.

Functions of Cytokines

Cytokines are crucial regulators of cells and hence control their growth, movement, evolution and differentiation. Being responsible for so many factors they are generated in response to varied stimuli. The most critical of these stimuli are antigen-antibody complexes acting through antibody receptors (FcRs), pathogen-associated molecular patterns (PAMPs) such as lipopolysaccharides acting through toll-like receptors (TLRs) and antigens acting through the B cell or T cell antigen receptors. Cytokines acts on different cells and in different ways. Cytokines may have an autocrine effect (Cytokines bind to receptors that produced them), paracrine effect (Cytokines bind to receptors on neighboring or cells which are very close) or endocrine effect (Cytokines flow throughout the body) while acting on the target cells. Cytokines also play role in apoptosis and control various stages of replication. They have the capability for being sensitive markers of chemically induced perturbations in function, but this claim is not accepted from the toxicological point of view. The reasons behind this being that cytokines are released locally with plasma measures being unreliable and they have short half-lives which need precise timing to find.

Cytokine structure

Cytokines have distinct structures but can be broadly divided into following.

Group I cytokines are involved in immune regulation --- includes four α -helices in bundles, Interferon subfamily and the IL-10 subfamily.

Group II cytokines are engaged in growth and regulation of cells, cell death and inflammation --- IL-1 family, TGF-β

Group III cytokines are involved in inflammation--- Chemokines

Group IV cytokines --- IL-12

Table: Different cytokines and their source:

Cytokine	Principal Cell Source
Interleukin-1 (IL -1)	Macrophages, endothelial cells, some epithelial cells
Interleukin-6 (IL -6)	Macrophages, endothelial cells, T cells
Interleukin-10 (IL-10)	Macrophages, T cells (mainly regulatory T cells)
Interleukin-12 (IL-12)	Macrophages, dendritic cells
Interleukin-15 (IL-15)	Macrophages, others
Interleukin-18 (IL-18)	Macrophages
Interleukin-23 (IL-23)	Macrophages and dendritic cells
Interleukin-27 (IL-27)	Macrophages and dendritic cells
Chemokines	Macrophages, endothelial cells, T cells, fibroblasts, platelets
Type I interferons (IFN -α, IFN-β)	IFN-α: macrophages; IFN-β: fibroblasts
Tumor necrosis factor (TNF)	Macrophages, T cells

Cytokine Receptor

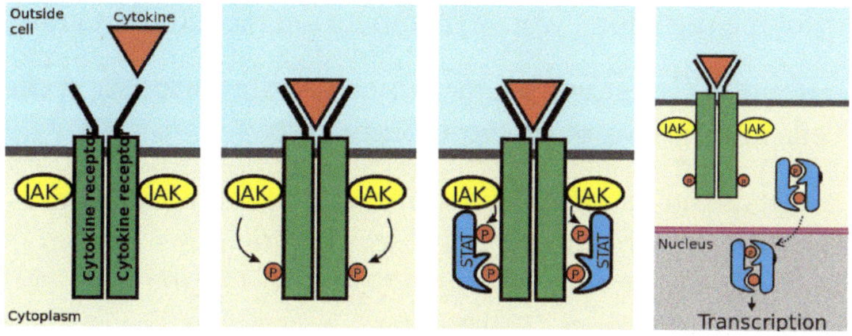

Key steps of the JAK-STAT pathway for type 1 and 2 cytokine receptors

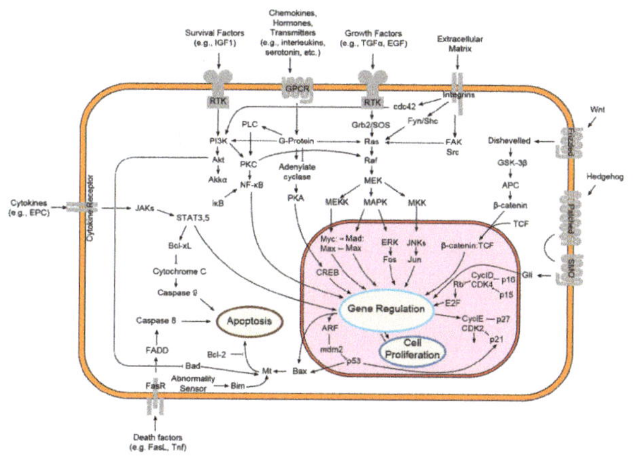

Signal transduction. (Cytokine receptor at center left.)

Cytokine receptors are receptors that bind cytokines.

In recent years, the cytokine receptors have come to demand the attention of more investigators than cytokines themselves, partly because of their remarkable characteristics, and partly because a deficiency of cytokine receptors has now been directly linked to certain debilitating immunodeficiency states. In this regard, and also because the redundancy and pleiotropy of cytokines are a consequence of their homologous receptors, many authorities are now of the opinion that a classification of cytokine receptors would be more clinically and experimentally useful.

Classification

A classification of cytokine receptors based on their three-dimensional structure has been attempted. (Such a classification, though seemingly cumbersome, provides several unique perspectives for attractive pharmacotherapeutic targets.)

- Type I cytokine receptors, whose members have certain conserved motifs in their extracellular amino-acid domain. The IL-2 receptor belongs to this chain, whose γ-chain (common to several other cytokines) deficiency is directly responsible for the x-linked form of Severe Combined Immunodeficiency (X-SCID).

- Type II cytokine receptors, whose members are receptors mainly for interferons.
- Immunoglobulin (Ig) superfamily, which are ubiquitously present throughout several cells and tissues of the vertebrate body
- Tumor necrosis factor receptor family, whose members share a cysteine-rich common extracellular binding domain, and includes several other non-cytokine ligands like receptors, CD40, CD27 and CD30, besides the ligands on which the family is named (TNF).
- Chemokine receptors, two of which acting as binding proteins for HIV (CXCR4 and CCR5). They are G protein coupled receptors.
- TGF beta receptors

Comparison

Type	Examples	Structure	Mechanism
type I cytokine receptor	• Type 1 interleukin receptors • Erythropoietin receptor • GM-CSF receptor • G-CSF receptor • growth hormone receptor • prolactin receptor • Oncostatin M receptor • Leukemia inhibitory factor receptor	Certain conserved motifs in their extracellular amino-acid domain. Connected to Janus kinase (JAK) family of tyrosine kinases	JAK phosphorylate and activate downstream proteins involved in their signal transduction pathways
type II cytokine receptor	• Type II interleukin receptors • interferon-alpha/beta receptor • interferon-gamma receptor		
Many members of the **immunoglobulin superfamily**	• Interleukin-1 receptor • CSF1 • C-kit receptor • Interleukin-18 receptor	Share structural homology with immunoglobulins (antibodies), cell adhesion molecules, and even some cytokines.	
Tumor necrosis factor receptor family	• CD27 • CD30 • CD40 • CD120 • Lymphotoxin beta receptor	cysteine-rich common extracellular binding domain	

chemokine receptors	• Interleukin-8 receptor • CCR1 • CXCR4 • MCAF receptor • NAP-2 receptor	Seven transmembrane helix	G protein-coupled
TGF beta receptors	• TGF beta receptor 1 • TGF beta receptor 2		

Solubility

Cytokine receptors may be both membrane-bound and soluble. *Soluble cytokine receptors* are extremely common regulators of cytokine function. Soluble cytokine receptors typically consist of the extracellular portions of membrane-bound receptors. .

Cytokine Regulation

The three major ways for regulating the cytokine signaling are –

- By specific binding proteins
- By changes in receptor expression and
- By cytokines that exert opposite effects.

Concept behind understanding the cytokine regulation is that as the single cell receives signals from numerous cytokine receptors, a unification of multiple signals is required to generate a coherent response.

Signal Transduction and Pathways

During the signal transduction the first step is the binding of cytokines to its receptors. Once the binding occurs, the receptor transmits a signal to the cell to alter its behavior. This phenomenon involving conversion of an extracellular signal into a series of intracellular events is called signal transduction. As Cell signaling needs to be precise and quick, enzyme cascade serve this function by the amplification of the responses rapidly. The important features of signal transduction include binding of cytokine to a cell surface receptor, stimulation of a transducer protein by the receptor, secondary activation of various enzymes, production of new transcription factors and ultimately gene stimulation leading to changed cell behavior.

Although there are many pathways of signal transduction but three pathways are of utmost significance to the immune system.

- The NF-kB pathway
- The NF-AT pathway
- The JAK/STAT pathway

The NF-κβ Pathway

NF-κβ has its origins in the family of five transcription factors that play a crucial role in inflammation and immunity. There are more than 150 genes that get expressed on NF-κβ stimulation. There are three major pathways for NF-κβ activation. These are the classical pathway , alternative pathway and the third pathway that is stimulated by DNA damaging drugs and Ultraviolet light. The classical pathway involves proinflammatory signaling and gets activated by inflammatory cytokines, TLRs and antigen receptors. IKK (Iκβ) complex is the central regulator of NF-κβ and all the signals induced by various stimuli focus on the same complex IKK. IKK complex is rich with kinase activity and on activation IKK complex phosphorylates Iκβ. Consequently Iκβ dissociates from the NF-κβ and the newly formed Iκβ becomes ubiquinated and is destroyed by proteasomes. Dissociation between Iκβ and NF-κβ liberates NF-κβ and it enters the nucleus to activate κβ motif containing promoters on DNA. This stimulates many genes and cytokines IL-1β, IL-6, IL-18, IL-33, TNF-α, GM-CSF, and IL-4. The second pathway or alternative pathway is required for lymphocyte development and is stimulated by a subset of TNF receptors. The third pathway does not require any IKK activation.

IKK- Iκβ kinase

Iκβ- Inhibitor of NF-κβ

NEMO- NF-κB essential modulator

TRAF- Tumor necrosis factor receptor-associated factor

Figure: NF-κβ signaling pathway:

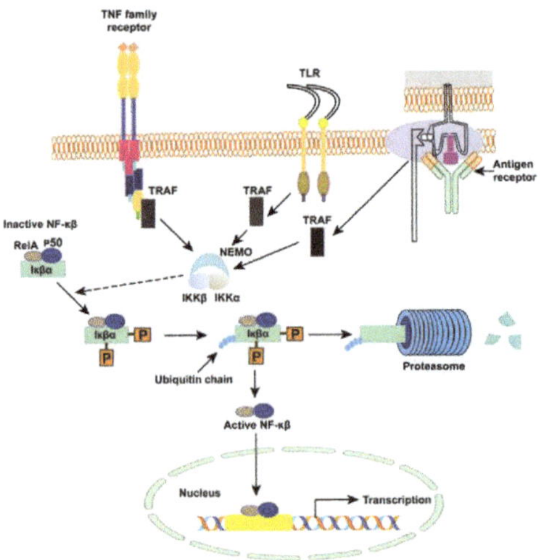

The NF-AT Pathway

The response generated to a T- cell is transmitted from the T cell receptor to a signal transducing complex called CD3 which is followed by clustering of CD3 chains in lipid rafts. Immunoreceptor tyrosine-based, activation motifs (ITAMs) are the specific amino acid sequences in the cytoplasmic domains of CD3 proteins. ITAMs later on become binding sites for several tyrosine kinases on activation. Zeta associated protein – 70 (ZAP-70) is one of the TKs and on phosphorylation can stimulate three signaling pathways. In the first pathway activation of calcineurin, a phosphatase is required and it ends up by generating NF-κβ and NF-AT . In the second pathway, ZAP-70 stimulates a protein kinase C which is required for activation of NF-κβ . The third pathway activates ras, a GTP-binding protein, fos and jun.

The JAK-STAT Pathway

More than 40 cytokines use the JAK-STAT pathway. The stimulated JAK (Janus kinase) molecules phosphorylate tyrosine residues on one of several STAT proteins (signal transducers and activators of transcription). Phosphorylated STAT proteins then dimerize and dissociate from JAK and get shifted to the nucleus where they regulate the expression of target genes.

Figure: JAK-STAT signaling pathway:

Cytokine ligation to cytokine receptor leads to activation of JAK tyrosine kinase, phosphorylation of its cytoplasmic domain, and recruitment of STAT. Recruitment of STAT and its phosphorylation dimerizes and transport it to nucleus. This event activates the transcription of cytokine gene.

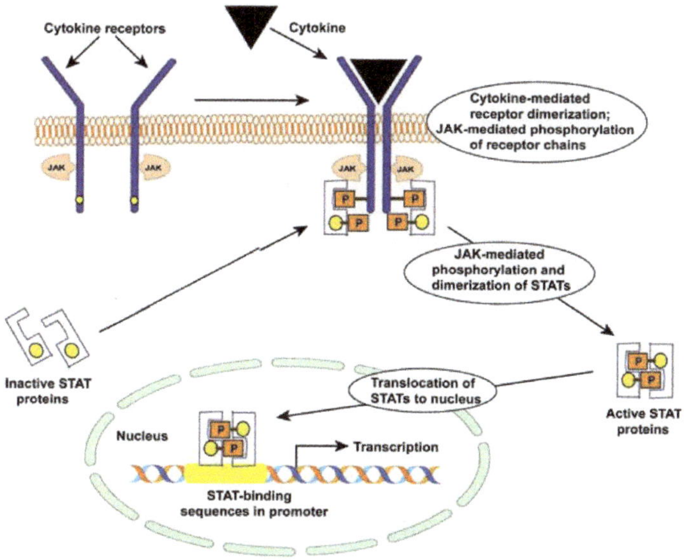

Interferon alpha/beta domain

Interferon

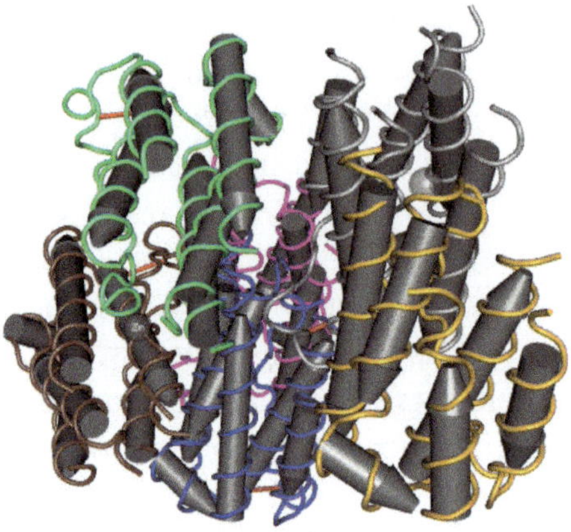

The molecular structure of human interferon-alpha

Interferons (IFNs) are a group of signaling proteins made and released by host cells in response to the presence of several pathogens, such as viruses, bacteria, parasites, and also tumor cells. In a typical scenario, a virus-infected cell will release interferons causing nearby cells to heighten their anti-viral defenses.

IFNs belong to the large class of proteins known as cytokines, molecules used for communication between cells to trigger the protective defenses of the immune system that help eradicate pathogens. Interferons are named for their ability to "interfere" with viral replication by protecting cells from virus infections. IFNs also have various other functions: they activate immune cells, such as natural killer cells and macrophages; they increase host defenses by up-regulating antigen presentation by virtue of increasing the expression of major histocompatibility complex (MHC) antigens. Certain symptoms of infections, such as fever, muscle pain and "flu-like symptoms", are also caused by the production of IFNs and other cytokines.

More than twenty distinct IFN genes and proteins have been identified in animals, including humans. They are typically divided among three classes: Type I IFN, Type II IFN, and Type III IFN. IFNs belonging to all three classes are important for fighting viral infections and for the regulation of the immune system.

Types of Interferon

Based on the type of receptor through which they signal, human interferons have been classified into three major types.

- Interferon type I: All type I IFNs bind to a specific cell surface receptor complex known as the IFN-α/β receptor (IFNAR) that consists of IFNAR1 and IFNAR2 chains. The type I interferons present in humans are IFN-α, IFN-β,

IFN-ε, IFN-κ and IFN-ω. In general, type I interferons are produced when the body recognizes a virus has invaded it. They are produced by fibroblasts and monocytes. However, the production of type I IFN-α is prohibited by another cytokine known as Interleukin-10. Once released, type I interferons will activate molecules which prevent the virus from producing and replicating its RNA and DNA. Overall, IFN-α can be used to treat hepatitis B and C infections, while IFN-β can be used to treat multiple sclerosis.

- Interferon type II (IFN-γ in humans): This is also known as immune interferon and is activated by Interleukin-12. Furthermore, type II interferons are released by T helper cells, type 1 specifically. However, they block the proliferation of T helper cells type two. The previous results in an inhibition of Th2 immune response and a further induction of Th1 immune response, which leads to the development of debilitating diseases such as multiple sclerosis. IFN type II binds to IFNGR, which consists of IFNGR1 and IFNGR2 chains and has a different receptor than type I IFN.
- Interferon type III: Signal through a receptor complex consisting of IL10R2 (also called CRF2-4) and IFNLR1 (also called CRF2-12). Although discovered more recently than type I and type II IFNs, recent information demonstrates the importance of Type III IFNs in some types of virus infections.

In general, type I and II interferons are responsible for regulating and activating the immune response. Expression of type I and III IFNs can be induced in virtually all cell types upon recognition of viral components, especially nucleic acids, by cytoplasmic and endosomal receptors, whereas type II interferon is induced by cytokines such as IL-12, and its expression is restricted to immune cells such as T cells and NK cells.

Function

All interferons share several common effects: they are antiviral agents and they modulate functions of the immune system. Administration of Type I IFN has been shown experimentally to inhibit tumor growth in animals, but the beneficial action in human tumors has not been widely documented. A virus-infected cell releases viral particles that can infect nearby cells. However, the infected cell can prepare neighboring cells against a potential infection by the virus by releasing interferons. In response to interferon, cells produce large amounts of an enzyme known as protein kinase R (PKR). This enzyme phosphorylates a protein known as eIF-2 in response to new viral infections; the phosphorylated eIF-2 forms an inactive complex with another protein, called eIF2B, to reduce protein synthesis within the cell. Another cellular enzyme, RNAse L—also induced by interferon action—destroys RNA within the cells to further reduce protein synthesis of both viral and host genes. Inhibited protein synthesis destroys both the virus and infected host cells. In addition, interferons induce production of hundreds of other proteins—known collectively as interferon-stimulated genes (ISGs)—that have roles in combating viruses and other actions produced by interferon. They also limit viral spread by increasing p53 activity, which kills virus-infected cells by promoting apoptosis. The effect of IFN on p53 is also linked to its protective role against certain cancers.

Another function of interferons is to upregulate major histocompatibility complex molecules, MHC I and MHC II, and increase immunoproteasome activity. Higher MHC I expression increases presentation of viral peptides to cytotoxic T cells, while the immunoproteasome processes viral peptides for loading onto the MHC I molecule, thereby increasing the recognition and killing of infected cells. Higher MHC II expression increases presentation of viral peptides to helper T cells; these cells release cytokines (such as more interferons and interleukins, among others) that signal to and co-ordinate the activity of other immune cells.

Interferons, such as interferon gamma, directly activate other immune cells, such as macrophages and natural killer cells.

Induction of Interferons

Production of interferons occurs mainly in response to microbes, such as viruses and bacteria, and their products. Binding of molecules uniquely found in microbes—viral glycoproteins, viral RNA, bacterial endotoxin (lipopolysaccharide), bacterial flagella, CpG motifs—by pattern recognition receptors, such as membrane bound Toll like receptors or the cytoplasmic receptors RIG-I or MDA5, can trigger release of IFNs. Toll Like Receptor 3 (TLR3) is important for inducing interferons in response to the presence of double-stranded RNA viruses; the ligand for this receptor is double-stranded RNA (dsRNA). After binding dsRNA, this receptor activates the transcription factors IRF3 and NF-κB, which are important for initiating synthesis of many inflammatory proteins. RNA interference technology tools such as siRNA or vector-based reagents can either silence or stimulate interferon pathways. Release of IFN from cells (specifically IFN-γ in lymphoid cells) is also induced by mitogens. Other cytokines, such as interleukin 1, interleukin 2, interleukin-12, tumor necrosis factor and colony-stimulating factor, can also enhance interferon production.

Downstream Signaling

By interacting with their specific receptors, IFNs activate *signal transducer and activator of transcription* (STAT) complexes; STATs are a family of transcription factors that regulate the expression of certain immune system genes. Some STATs are activated by both type I and type II IFNs. However each IFN type can also activate unique STATs.

STAT activation initiates the most well-defined cell signaling pathway for all IFNs, the classical Janus kinase-STAT (JAK-STAT) signaling pathway. In this pathway, JAKs associate with IFN receptors and, following receptor engagement with IFN, phosphorylate both STAT1 and STAT2. As a result, an IFN-stimulated gene factor 3 (ISGF3) complex forms—this contains STAT1, STAT2 and a third transcription factor called IRF9—and moves into the cell nucleus. Inside the nucleus, the ISGF3 complex binds to specific nucleotide sequences called *IFN-stimulated response elements* (ISREs) in the promoters of certain genes, known as IFN stimulated genes ISGs. Binding of ISGF3 and other transcriptional complexes activated by IFN signaling to these specific regulatory elements induces transcription of those genes. A collection of known ISGs is available on Interferome, a curated online database of ISGs; Additionally, STAT homodimers or heterodimers form from different combinations of STAT-1, -3, -4, -5, or -6 during IFN signaling; these dimers initiate gene transcription by binding to IFN-activated site (GAS) elements in gene promoters. Type I IFNs can induce expression of genes with either ISRE or GAS elements, but gene induction by type II IFN can occur only in the presence of a GAS element.

In addition to the JAK-STAT pathway, IFNs can activate several other signaling cascades. For instance, both type I and type II IFNs activate a member of the CRK family of adaptor proteins called CRKL, a nuclear adaptor for STAT5 that also regulates signaling through the C3G/Rap1 pathway. Type I IFNs further activate *p38 mitogen-activated protein kinase* (MAP kinase) to induce gene transcription. Antiviral and antiproliferative effects specific to type I IFNs result from p38 MAP kinase signaling. The *phosphatidylinositol 3-kinase* (PI3K) signaling pathway is also regulated by both type I and type II IFNs. PI3K activates P70-S6 Kinase 1, an enzyme that increases protein synthesis and cell proliferation; phosphorylates of ribosomal protein s6, which is involved in protein synthesis; and phosphorylates a translational repressor protein called *eukaryotic translation-initiation factor 4E-binding protein 1* (EIF4EBP1) in order to deactivate it.

Virus Resistance to Interferons

Many viruses have evolved mechanisms to resist interferon activity. They circumvent the IFN response by blocking downstream signaling events that occur after the cytokine binds to its receptor, by preventing further IFN production, and by inhibiting the functions of proteins that are induced by IFN. Viruses that inhibit IFN signaling include Japanese Encephalitis Virus (JEV), dengue type 2 virus (DEN-2) and viruses of the herpesvirus family, such as human cytomegalovirus (HCMV) and Kaposi's sarcoma-associated herpesvirus (KSHV or HHV8). Viral proteins proven to affect IFN signaling include EBV nuclear antigen 1 (EBNA1) and EBV nuclear antigen 2 (EBNA-2) from Epstein-Barr virus, the large T antigen of Polyomavirus, the E7 protein of Human papillomavirus (HPV), and the B18R protein of vaccinia virus. Reducing IFN-α activity may prevent signaling via STAT1, STAT2, or IRF9 (as with JEV infection) or through the JAK-STAT pathway (as with DEN-2 infection). Several poxviruses encode soluble IFN receptor homologs—like the B18R protein of the vaccinia virus—that bind to and prevent IFN interacting with its cellular receptor, impeding communication between this cytokine and its target cells. Some viruses can encode proteins that bind to double-stranded RNA (dsRNA) to prevent the activity of RNA-dependent protein kinases; this is the mechanism reovirus adopts using its sigma 3 (σ3) protein, and vaccinia virus employs using the gene product of its E3L gene, p25. The ability of interferon to induce protein production from interferon stimulated genes (ISGs) can also be affected. Production of protein kinase R, for example, can be disrupted in cells infected with JEV Some viruses escape the anti-viral activities of interferons by gene (and thus protein) mutation. The H5N1 influenza virus, also known as bird flu, has resistance to interferon and other anti-viral cytokines that is attributed to a single amino acid change in its Non-Structural Protein 1 (NS1), although the precise mechanism of how this confers immunity is unclear.

Interferon Therapy

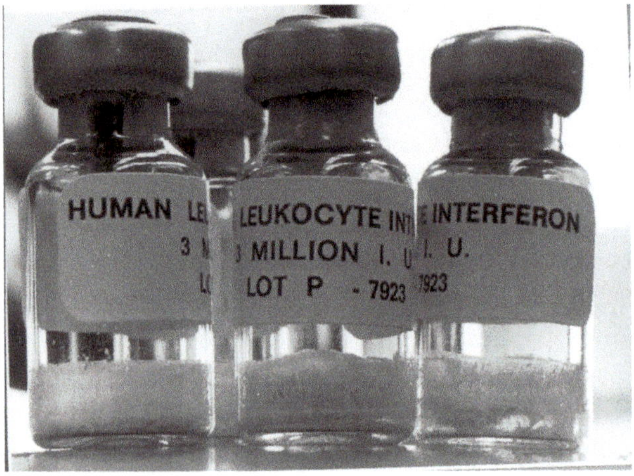

Three vials filled with human leukocyte interferon

Diseases

Interferon beta-1a and interferon beta-1b are used to treat and control multiple sclerosis, an autoimmune disorder. This treatment is effective for reducing attacks in relapsing-remitting multiple sclerosis and slowing disease progression and activity in secondary progressive multiple sclerosis.

Interferon therapy is used (in combination with chemotherapy and radiation) as a treatment for some cancers. This treatment can be used in hematological malignancy; leukemia and lymphomas including hairy cell leukemia, chronic myeloid leukemia, nodular lymphoma, and cutaneous T-cell lymphoma. Patients with recurrent melanomas receive recombinant IFN-α2b. Both hepatitis B and hepatitis C are treated with IFN-α, often in combination with other antiviral drugs. Some of those treated with interferon have a sustained virological response and can eliminate hepatitis virus. The most harmful strain—hepatitis C genotype I virus—can be treated with a 60-80% success rate with the current standard-of-care treatment of interferon-α, ribavirin and recently approved protease inhibitors such as Telaprevir (Incivek) May 2011, Boceprevir (Victrelis) May 2011 or the nucleotide analog polymerase inhibitor Sofosbuvir (Sovaldi) December 2013. Biopsies of patients given the treatment show reductions in liver damage and cirrhosis. Some evidence shows giving interferon immediately following infection can prevent chronic hepatitis C, although diagnosis early in infection is difficult since physical symptoms are sparse in early hepatitis C infection. Control of chronic hepatitis C by IFN is associated with reduced hepatocellular carcinoma.

Interferon treatment was evaluated in individuals suffering from herpes simplex virus epithelial keratitis. Topical interferon therapy was shown to be an effective treatment, especially with higher concentrations. Interferon, either used alone or in combination with debridement, appears to be as effective as a nucleoside antiviral agent. The combination of interferon and another nucleoside antiviral agent may speed the healing process.

When used in the systemic therapy, IFNs are mostly administered by an intramuscular injection. The injection of IFNs in the muscle or under skin is generally well tolerated. The most frequent adverse effects are flu-like symptoms: increased body temperature, feeling ill, fatigue, headache, muscle pain, convulsion, dizziness, hair thinning, and depression. Erythema, pain and hardness on the spot of injection are also frequently observed. IFN therapy causes immunosuppression, in particular through neutropenia and can result in some infections manifesting in unusual ways.

Drug formulations

Pharmaceutical forms of interferons	
Generic name	**Trade name**
Interferon alpha 2a	Roferon A
Interferon alpha 2b	Intron A/Reliferon/Uniferon
Human leukocyte Interferon-alpha (HuIFN-alpha-Le)	Multiferon
Interferon beta 1a, liquid form	Rebif
Interferon beta 1a, lyophilized	Avonex
Interferon beta 1a, biogeneric (Iran)	Cinnovex
Interferon beta 1b	Betaseron / Betaferon
Interferon gamma 1b	Actimmune
PEGylated interferon alpha 2a	Pegasys
PEGylated interferon alpha 2a (Egypt)	Reiferon Retard
PEGylated interferon alpha 2b	PegIntron
PEGylated interferon alpha 2b plus ribavirin (Canada)	Pegetron

Several different types of interferons are approved for use in humans. One was first approved for medical use in 1986. For example, in January 2001, the Food and Drug Administration (FDA) approved the use of PEGylated interferon-alpha in the USA; in this formulation, PEGylated interferon-alpha-2b (*Pegintron*), polyethylene glycol is linked to the interferon molecule to make the interferon last longer in the body. Approval for PEGylated interferon-alpha-2a (*Pegasys*) followed in October 2002. These PEGylated drugs are injected once weekly, rather than administering two or three times per week, as is necessary for conventional interferon-alpha. When used with the antiviral drug ribavirin, PEGylated interferon is effective in treatment of hepatitis C; at least 75% of people with hepatitis C genotypes 2 or 3 benefit from interferon treatment, although this is effective in less than 50% of people infected with genotype 1 (the more common form of hepatitis C virus in both the U.S. and Western Europe). Interferon-containing regimens may also include protease inhibitors such as boceprevir and telaprevir.

History

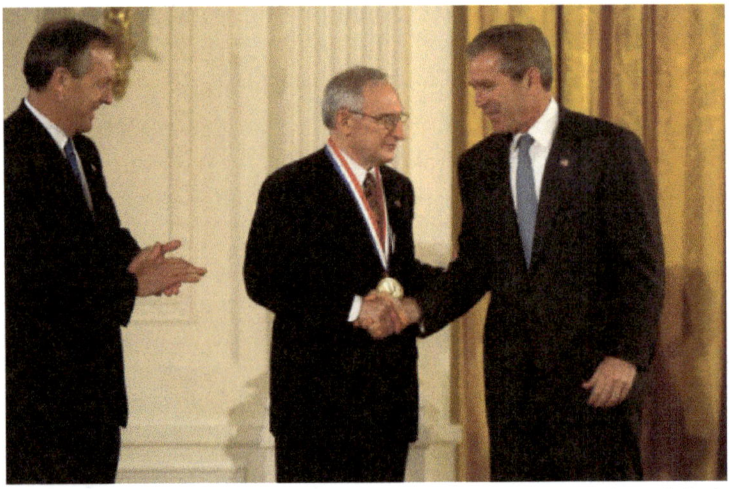

Sidney Pestka of Rutgers University, seen here receiving the National Medal of Technology.

Interferons were first described in 1957 by Alick Isaacs and Jean Lindenmann at the National Institute for Medical Research in London; the discovery was a result of their studies of viral interference. Viral interference refers to the inhibition of virus growth caused by previous exposure of cells to an active or a heat-inactivated virus. Isaacs and Lindenmann were working with a system that involved the inhibition of the growth of live influenza virus in chicken embryo chorioallantoic membranes by heat-inactivated influenza virus. Their experiments revealed that this interference was mediated by a protein released by cells in the heat-inactivated influenza virus-treated membranes. They published their results in 1957 naming the antiviral factor they had discovered *interferon*. The findings of Isaacs and Lindenmann have been widely confirmed and corroborated in the literature.

Furthermore, others may have made observations on interferons before the publication of Isaacs and Lindenmann. For example, during research to produce a more efficient vaccine for smallpox, Yasu-ichi Nagano and Yasuhiko Kojima—two Japanese virologists working at the Institute for Infectious Diseases at the University of Tokyo—noticed inhibition of viral growth in an area of rabbit-skin or testis previously inoculated with UV-inactivated virus. They hypothesised that some "viral inhibitory factor" was present in the tissues infected with virus and attempted to isolate and characterize this factor from tissue homogenates. Independently, Monto Ho, in John Enders's lab, observed in 1957 that attenuated poliovirus conferred a species specific anti-viral effect in human amniotic cell cultures. They described these observations in a publication, naming the responsible factor *viral inhibitory factor* (VIF). It took another fifteen to twenty years, using somatic cell genetics, to show that the interferon action gene and interferon gene reside in different human chromosomes. The purification of human beta interferon did not occur until 1977. Chris Y.H. Tan and his co-workers purified and produced biologically active, radio-labeled human beta interferon by superinducing the interferon gene in fibroblast cells, and they showed its active site contains tyrosine residues. Tan's laboratory isolated sufficient amounts of human beta interferon to perform the first amino acid, sugar composition and N-terminal analyses. They showed that human beta interferon was an unusually hydrophobic glycoprotein. This explained the large loss of interferon activity when preparations were transferred from test tube to test tube or from vessel to vessel during purification. The analyses showed the reality of interferon activity by chemical verification. The purification of human alpha interferon was not reported until 1978. A series of publications from the laboratories of Sidney Pestka and Alan Waldman between 1978 and 1981, describe the purification of the type I interferons IFN-α and IFN-β. By the early 1980s, genes for these interferons had been cloned, adding further definitive proof that interferons were responsible for interfering with viral replication. Gene cloning also confirmed that IFN-α was encoded by a family of many related genes. The type II IFN (IFN-γ) gene was also isolated around this time.

Interferon was scarce and expensive until 1980, when the interferon gene was inserted into bacteria using recombinant DNA technology, allowing mass cultivation and purification from bacterial cultures or derived from yeasts. Interferon can also be produced by recombinant mammalian cells. Before the early 1970s, large scale production of human interferon had been pioneered by Kari Cantell. He produced large amounts of human alpha interferon from large quantities of human white blood cells collected by the Finnish Blood Bank. Large amounts of human beta interferon were made by superinducing the beta interferon gene in human fibroblast cells.

Cantell's and Tan's methods of making large amounts of natural interferon were critical for chemical characterisation, clinical trials and the preparation of small amounts of interferon messenger RNA to clone the human alpha and beta interferon genes. The superinduced human beta interferon messenger RNA was prepared by Tan's lab for Cetus corp. to clone the human beta interferon gene in bacteria and the recombinant interferon was developed as 'betaseron' and approved for the treatment of MS. Superinduction of the human beta interferon gene was also used by Israeli scientists to manufacture human beta interferon.

Human Interferons

- IFNA1
- IFNA2
- IFNA4
- IFNA5
- IFNA6
- IFNA7
- IFNA8
- IFNA10
- IFNA13
- IFNA14
- IFNA16
- IFNA17
- IFNA21
- IFNB1
- IFNW
- IFNE1
- IFNK

References

- "Revised nomenclature for antigen-nonspecific T cell proliferation and helper factors". Journal of Immunology. 123 (6): 2928–9. Dec 1979. PMID 91646
- James, William; Berger, Timothy; Elston, Dirk (2005). Andrews' Diseases of the Skin: Clinical Dermatology. (10th ed.). Saunders. ISBN 0-7216-2921-0
- Noosheen Alaverdi; David Sehy (2007-05-01). "Cytokines - Master Regulators of the Immune System" (PDF). eBioscience. Retrieved 2008-02-28
- Leng SX, Elias JA (1997). "Interleukin-11". The International Journal of Biochemistry & Cell Biology. 29 (8-9): 1059–62. doi:10.1016/S1357-2725(97)00017-4. PMID 9416001
- Julius M. Cruse; Robert Edwin Lewis (20 April 2009). Illustrated dictionary of immunology. CRC Press. pp. 208–. ISBN 978-0-8493-7987-1. Retrieved 24 April 2011
- Royal Swedish Academy of Sciences (10 October 2012). "The Nobel Prize in Chemistry 2012 Robert J. Lefkowitz, Brian K. Kobilka". Retrieved 10 October 2012

- Park AY, Scott P (Jun 2001). “Il-12: keeping cell-mediated immunity alive”. Scandinavian Journal of Immunology. 53 (6): 529–32. doi:10.1046/j.1365-3083.2001.00917.x. PMID 11422900
- Schindler R, Dinarello CA (1990). “Interleukin 1”. In Habenicht A. Growth Factors, Differentiation Factors, and Cytokines. Berlin, Heidelberg: Springer. doi:10.1007/978-3-642-74856-1_7. ISBN 978-3-642-74856-1
- “The Top Prescription Drugs of 2012 Globally: Biologics Dominate, But Small Molecule CNS Drugs Hold on to Top Spots” (PDF). ACS Chemical Neuroscience. Retrieved 2016-02-03
- Abbas AK, Lichtman AH, Pillai S (2012). Cellular and molecular immunology (7th ed.). Philadelphia: Elsevier/Saunders. ISBN 1437715281
- Kolata, Gina (2015-01-22). “Jean Lindenmann, Who Made Interferon His Life’s Work, Is Dead at 90”. New York Times. Retrieved 2015-02-12
- Aggarwal S, Gurney AL (Jan 2002). “IL-17: prototype member of an emerging cytokine family”. Journal of Leukocyte Biology. 71 (1): 1–8. PMID 11781375
- Long, Sarah S.; Pickering, Larry K.; Prober, Charles G. (2012). Principles and Practice of Pediatric Infectious Disease. Elsevier Health Sciences. p. 1502. ISBN 1437727026
- Mélik-Parsadaniantz, Stéphane; Rostène, William (2008). “Chemokines and neuromodulation”. Journal of Neuroimmunology. 198 (1–2): 62–8. doi:10.1016/j.jneuroim.2008.04.022. PMID 18538863
- Heaney ML1, Golde DW (1998). “Soluble receptors in human disease”. Journal of Leukocyte Biology. 64 (2): 135–146. PMID 9715251
- Goldstein D, Laszlo J (Sep 1988). “The role of interferon in cancer therapy: a current perspective” (Free full text). CA: A Cancer Journal for Clinicians. 38 (5): 258–277. doi:10.3322/canjclin.38.5.258. PMID 2458171
- Cantell K (1998). The story of interferon: the ups and downs in the life of a scientis. Singapore ; New York: World Scientific. ISBN 978-981-02-3148-4

5

Mechanism of Immune Response

The immune mechanism, to eradicate foreign substances or toxic microbes, are classified into humoral immunity and cellular immunity. The chapter also focuses on the functioning of participating Th17 cells and CD8+ cytotoxic T lymphocyte, etc. among other related topics. This section discusses the mechanism of immune response in a critical manner providing key analysis to the subject matter.

Leukocyte

The recruitment of the leukocyte and its activation is largely governed by the subset of CD4+ cells. Each leukocyte is specified for certain job and the cooperation of leukocyte to the lymphocytes is an important connection between innate and adaptive immune response.

In general Th1 cells activate macrophages, Th2 activates eosinophils, and Th17 activates neutrophils. The Th1 cells activate the macrophage mediated phagocytosis, Th2 stimulates the production of IgE in response to a helminthic infection, and Th17 activates neutrophils to extracellular microbes including bacteria and fungi. Cytotoxic T lymphocytes (CTLs) kill the microbes which escape the phagocytosis and replicate in the cytoplasm.

Migration of Lymphocyte at the Site of Infection

Majority of the leukocyte and lymphocyte are migrated towards the site of inflammation and infection, respectively in order to nullify the effect. Once the naïve lymphocyte encounters an antigen presented by the MHC molecule over the antigen presenting cells, they differentiate and migrate as an effector cells through the blood vessels to different parts of the body. The migration of lymphocyte is an interesting phenomenon orchestrated by different cytokines and specific receptors present over the surface of the lymphocytes. Naïve T lymphocytes express L-selectin and chemokine receptor CCR7 which help them to adhere to the lymph node and its surrounding tissues. After antigen stimulation the naïve T lymphocyte decrease the expression of L-selectin and CCR7 and increase the expression of sphingosine 1-phosphate receptors (S1PR1) , which help their migration into the blood vessels. Th1 cells produces large amount of ligands that binds to E and P-selectin which recognize selectins secreted at the site of bacterial infection and trigger a strong innate immune response. Th2 cells express different chemokine receptors such as CCR3, CCR4 and CCR8 which recognize specific Chemokines secreted at the site of helminthic infection. Similarly, Th17 migration to the site of fungal and bacterial infection is modulated by CCR6 and other cytokines. Usually the subset of T lymphocytes is directed to the site of action with the help of different chemokines and their respective ligands. Similarly memory cells express different integrins that binds to the fibronectins over the extracellular matrices and help in their migration.

Functions of CD4+ helper cells

The function of CD4+ cells are divided into four distinct stages.

- Leukocyte recruitment - T lymphocytes produces many cytokines that helps in the recruitment of neutrophils, eosinophils and monocytes at the site of infection or injury.
- Leukocyte activation - Leukocytes gets activated by the binding of CD40L on lymphocyte to the CD40 express over the antigen presenting cells.
- Expansion- The activation response gets expanded by the secretion of cytokines by the T lymphocytes.
- Control- The response of the immune system is controlled by some inhibitory cytokines such as IL-10.

T Helper Cell

Naïve T cells after encountering an MHC loaded peptide over the antigen presenting cells differentiates into Th1 cells. Th1 cells secretes interferon-γ (IFN-γ) which is a key cytokine involve in its functioning. IFN-γ acts on the activated macrophages and increases its phagocytosis efficiency and microbial killing. In addition IFN-γ also stimulates the B cells to secrete the IgG antibody that helps in opsonization and activation of complement pathway. Occasionally they also produce tumor necrosis factor that activate the neutrophils and promotes inflammation.

Functions of Th1 cells:

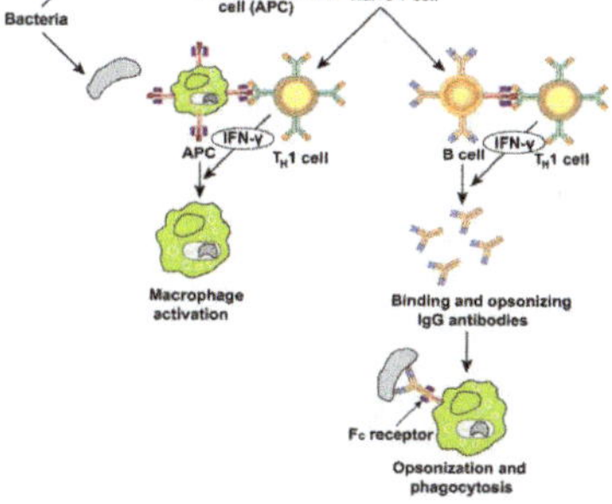

Function of Th17 Cells

After differentiation of naïve T cells into Th17 effector cells, they start secreting IL-17 and IL-22. IL-17 is a unique cytokine that do not have any homologue in the body. IL-17 stimulates the production of chemokines, TNF, IL-1, IL-6, and granulocyte-colony stimulating factors (G-CSF) which take part in inflammatory reactions. In addition, it is also involved in the production of defensins from the epithelial surface which in turn acts as a barrier for the invading pathogens. IL-22 is a relatively new interleukin and its function is not well established. However IL-22 is known to maintain the epithelial integrity, increase barrier function and involve in the repair activity following inflammation.

Figure: Functions of Th17 cells:

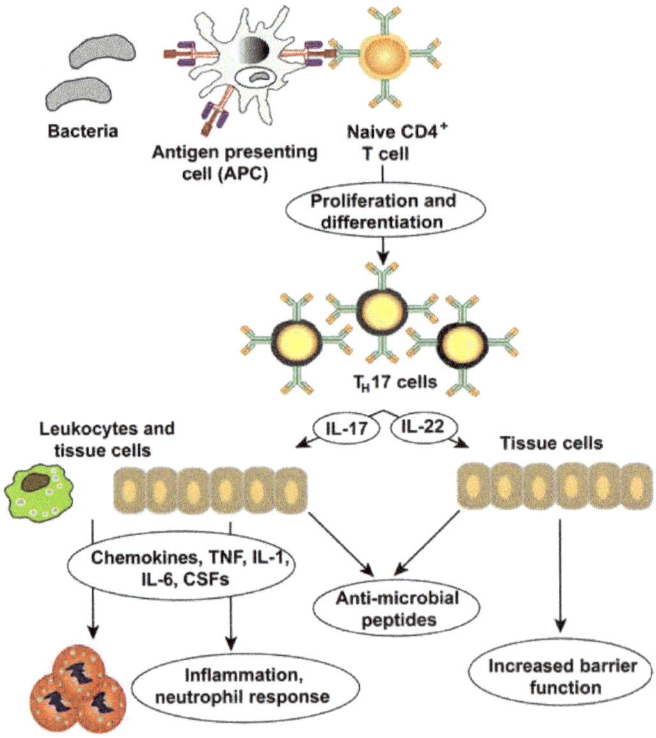

Function of CD8+ Cytotoxic T Lymphocyte

Cytotoxic T lymphocytes (CTLs) get activated after antigenic recognition over the MHC in the antigen presenting cells. The costimulatory molecules and their close association with other receptors results in the formation of immunological synapse (ICAM-1 to LFA-1). Activated CTLs secrete cytotoxic granules such as granzyme and perforin. Perforin is homologue to complement protein-9 and is known to produce holes and perforation in the target cell. Perforin polymerize to form an aqueous pore in the target cells through which granzyme enters the target cells. Granzyme is serine proteases which is responsible for the cleavage and activation of caspase in the cells leading to the apoptosis of the target cells. In addition, activated CTLs also secrete granules such as serglycin which are known to assemble the granzyme and perforin over the surface of target cells.

CTLs also kill the target cells in granule independent fashion by Fas Ligand mediated pathway. The Fas ligand binds to the death receptors that are expressed in many cell types and activates the caspase mediated apoptosis pathway.

The infection of intracellular microbes to host needs participation of CTLs because it will eliminate the reservoir of infection by killing the infected cell. Hepatitis B and C virus infection to a host activates the CTLs in order to kill the liver cells to eliminate the reservoir.

γδ T Cells

These are clonally distinct cells containing heterodimer of γ and δ chains, which are homologous to αand β chains in αβ T cells. Usually less than 5% of total circulating lymphocytes are composed of γδ T cell receptor. The γδ T cells present in the epithelial surface of bowel are called as intraepithelial lymphocytes . The γδ T cells do not recognize the MHC loaded peptide and are MHC independent. They require protein and non-proteinous antigen that do not require processing by MHC molecules.

Natural Killer Cells

T cells population that express the CD56 marker over their surface are called natural killer or NK cells. NK cells recognizes the lipid bound to CD1 receptor (MHC class I homologue). NK cell secretes IL-4 and interferon-γ after activation and help in the production of antibody by B cells. NK cell plays an important role in the protection against mycobacterium infection.

Points to Remember

- Cell mediated immunity is a type of adaptive immune response that is stimulated by microbes and can be transferred to naïve animal by T cells.
- Differentiation and migration of lymphocytes are orchestrated by different cytokines.
- Both CD4+ and CD8+ cells are responsible for cell mediated immunity
- CD4+ cells are comprised of Th1, Th2, and Th17 subsets and have different effector functions.
- CD8+ cells are converted into cytotoxic T lymphocyte upon differentiation and help in eradication of infection by killing the target cells.

Humoral Immunity

Humoral immunity or humoural immunity is the aspect of immunity that is mediated by macromolecules found in extracellular fluids such as secreted antibodies, complement proteins, and certain antimicrobial peptides. Humoral immunity is so named because it involves substances found in the humors, or body fluids. It contrasts with cell-mediated immunity. Its aspects involving antibodies are often called antibody-mediated immunity.

The study of the molecular and cellular components that form the immune system, including their function and interaction, is the central science of immunology. The immune system is divided into a more primitive innate immune system, and acquired or adaptive immune system of vertebrates, each of which contains humoral and cellular components.

Humoral immunity refers to antibody production and the accessory processes that accompany it, including: Th2 activation and cytokine production, germinal center formation and isotype switching, affinity maturation and memory cell generation. It also refers to the effector functions of antibodies, which include pathogen and toxin neutralization, classical complement activation, and opsonin promotion of phagocytosis and pathogen elimination.

History

The concept of humoral immunity developed based on analysis of antibacterial activity of the serum components. Hans Buchner is credited with the development of the humoral theory. In 1890 he described alexins, or "protective substances", which exist in the blood serum and other bodily fluid and are capable of killing microorganisms. Alexins, later redefined "complement" by Paul Ehrlich, were shown to be the soluble components of the innate response that lead to a combination of cellular and humoral immunity, and bridged the features of innate and acquired immunity.

Following the 1888 discovery of the bacteria that cause diphtheria and tetanus, Emil von Behring and Kitasato Shibasaburō showed that disease need not be caused by microorganisms themselves. They discovered that cell-free filtrates were sufficient to cause disease. In 1890, filtrates of diphtheria, later named diphtheria toxins, were used to vaccinate animals in an attempt to demonstrate that immunized serum contained an antitoxin that could neutralize the activity of the toxin and could transfer immunity to non-immune animals. In 1897, Paul Ehrlich showed that antibodies form against the plant toxins ricin and abrin, and proposed that these antibodies are responsible for immunity. Ehrlich, with his friend Emil von Behring, went on to develop the diphtheria antitoxin, which became the first major success of modern immunotherapy. The presence and specificity of compatibility antibodies became the major tool for standardizing the state of immunity and identifying the presence of previous infections.

Major discoveries in the study of humoral immunity		
Substance	**Activity**	**Discovery**
Alexin(s) Complement	Soluble components in the serum that are capable of killing microorganisms	Buchner (1890), Ehrlich (1892)
Antitoxins	Substances in the serum that can neutralize the activity of toxins, enabling passive immunization	von Behring and Kitasato (1890)
Bacteriolysins	Serum substances that work with the complement proteins to induce bacterial lysis	Richard Pfeiffer (1895)
Bacterial agglutinins and precipitins	Serum substances that agglutinate bacteria and precipitate bacterial toxins	von Gruber and Durham (1896), Kraus (1897)
Hemolysins	Serum substances that work with complement to lyse red blood cells	Belfanti and Carbone (1898) Jules Bordet (1899)
Opsonins	Serum substances that coat the outer membrane of foreign substances and enhance the rate of phagocytosis by macrophages	Wright and Douglas (1903)
Antibody	Formation (1900), antigen-antibody binding hypothesis (1938), produced by B cells (1948), structure (1972), immunoglobulin genes (1976)	Founder: P Ehrlich

Complement System

The complement system is a biochemical cascade of the innate immune system that helps clear pathogens from an organism. It is derived from many small blood plasma proteins that work together to disrupt the target cell's plasma membrane leading to cytolysis of the cell. The complement system consists of more than 35 soluble and cell-bound proteins, 12 of which are directly involved in the complement pathways. The complement system is involved in the activities of both innate immunity and acquired immunity.

Activation of this system leads to cytolysis, chemotaxis, opsonization, immune clearance, and inflammation, as well as the marking of pathogens for phagocytosis. The proteins account for 5% of the serum globulin fraction. Most of these proteins circulate as zymogens, which are inactive until proteolytic cleavage.

Three biochemical pathways activate the complement system: the classical complement pathway, the alternate complement pathway, and the mannose-binding lectin pathway. The classical complement pathway typically requires antibodies for activation and is a specific immune response, while the alternate pathway can be activated without the presence of antibodies and is considered a non-specific immune response. Antibodies, in particular the IgG1 class, can also "fix" complement.

B Cells

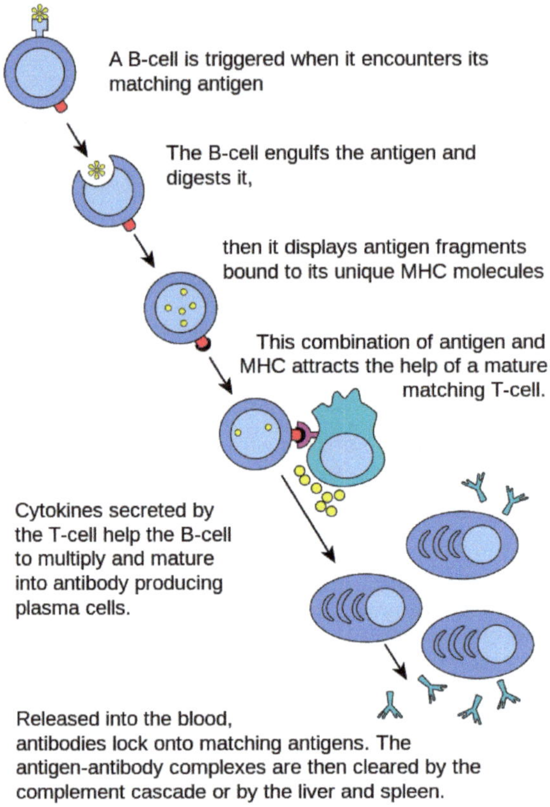

B cell activation is a large part of the humoral immune response.

The principal function of B cells is to make antibodies against soluble antigens. B cell recognition of antigen is not the only element necessary for B cell activation (a combination of clonal proliferation and the terminal differentiation into plasma cells).

Naïve B cells can be activated in a T-cell dependent or independent manner, but two signals are always required to initiate activation.

B cell activation depends on one of three mechanisms: *Type 1 T cell-independent* (polyclonal) activation, *Type 2 T cell-independent* activation (in which mature B cells respond to highly repetitive structures causing cross-linking of the B cell receptors on the surface of B cells), and T cell-dependent activation. During T cell-dependent activation, an antigen presenting cell (APC) presents a processed antigen to a T helper cell (T_h), priming it. When a B cell processes and presents the *same* antigen to the *primed T_h cell*, the T cell releases cytokines that activate the B cell.

Antibodies

Immunoglobulins are glycoproteins in the immunoglobulin superfamily that function as antibodies. The terms *antibody* and *immunoglobulin* are often used interchangeably. They are found in the blood and tissue fluids, as well as many secretions. In structure, they are large Y-shaped globular proteins. In mammals there are five types of antibody: IgA, IgD, IgE, IgG, and IgM. Each immunoglobulin class differs in its biological properties and has evolved to deal with different antigens. Antibodies are synthesized and secreted by plasma cells that are derived from the B cells of the immune system.

An antibody is used by the acquired immune system to identify and neutralize foreign objects like bacteria and viruses. Each antibody recognizes a specific antigen unique to its target. By binding their specific antigens, antibodies can cause agglutination and precipitation of antibody-antigen products, prime for phagocytosis by macrophages and other cells, block viral receptors, and stimulate other immune responses, such as the complement pathway.

An incompatible blood transfusion causes a transfusion reaction, which is mediated by the humoral immune response. This type of reaction, called an acute hemolytic reaction, results in the rapid destruction (hemolysis) of the donor red blood cells by host antibodies. The cause is usually a clerical error, such as the wrong unit of blood being given to the wrong patient. The symptoms are fever and chills, sometimes with back pain and pink or red urine (hemoglobinuria). The major complication is that hemoglobin released by the destruction of red blood cells can cause acute renal failure.

B cells, also known as B lymphocytes, are a type of white blood cell of the lymphocyte subtype. They function in the humoral immunity component of the adaptive immune system by secreting antibodies. Additionally, B cells present antigen (they are also classified as professional antigen-presenting cells (APCs)) and secrete cytokines.

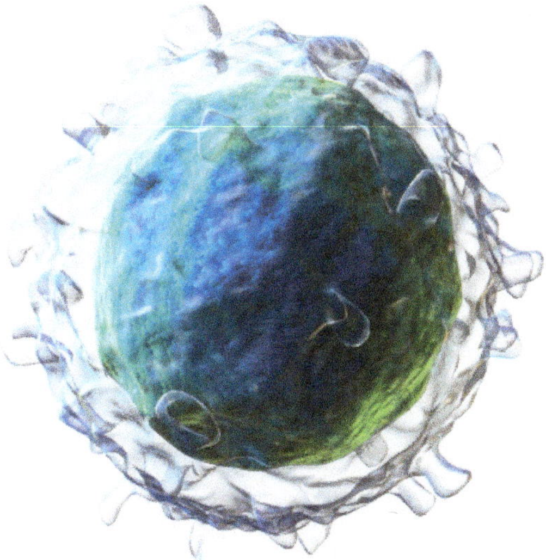

3D rendering of a B cell

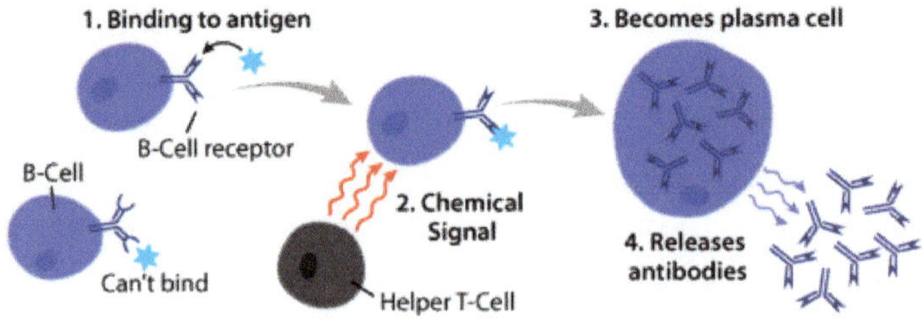

Basic B cell function: bind an antigen, receive help from a cognate helper T cell, and differentiate into a plasma cell that secretes large amounts of antibodies

In mammals, B cells mature in the bone marrow, which is at the core of most bones. In birds, B cells mature in the bursa of Fabricius, a lymphoid organ. (The "B" from B cells comes from the name of this organ, where it was first discovered by Chang and Glick, and not from bone marrow as commonly believed).

B cells, unlike the other two classes of lymphocytes, T cells and natural killer cells, express B cell receptors (BCRs) on their cell membrane. BCRs allow the B cell to bind a specific antigen, against which it will initiate an antibody response.

Development

B cells develop from hematopoietic stem cells (HSCs) that originate from bone marrow. HSCs first differentiate into multipotent progenitor (MPP) cells, then common lymphoid progenitor (CLP) cells. From here, their development into B cells occurs in several stages (shown in image to the right), each marked by various gene expression patterns and immunoglobulin H chain and L chain gene loci arrangements, the latter due to B cells undergoing V(D)J recombination as they develop.

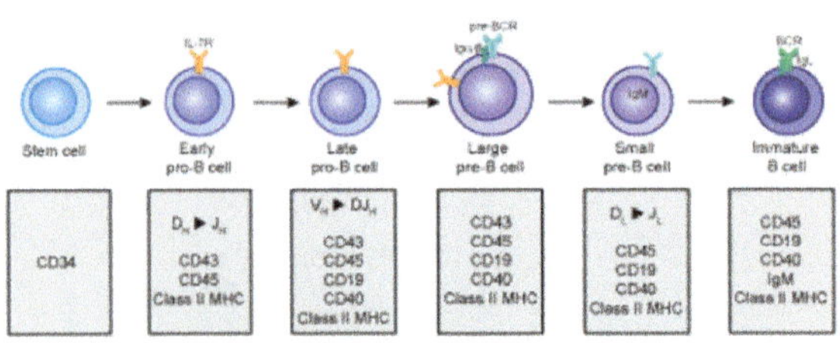

Early B cell development: from stem cell to immature B cell

B cells undergo two types of selection while developing in the bone marrow to ensure proper development. Positive selection occurs through antigen-independent signaling involving both the pre-BCR and the BCR. If these receptors do not bind to their ligand, B cells do not receive the proper signals and cease to develop. Negative selection occurs through the binding of self-antigen with the BCR; If the BCR can bind strongly to self-antigen, then the B cell undergoes one of four fates: clonal deletion, receptor editing, anergy, or ignorance (B cell ignores signal and continues development). This negative selection process leads to a state of central tolerance, in which the mature B cells don't bind with self antigens present in the bone marrow.

To complete development, immature B cells migrate from the bone marrow to the spleen as well as pass through two transitional stages: T1 and T2. Throughout their migration to the spleen and after spleen entry, they are considered T1 B cells. Within the spleen, T1 B cells transition to T2 B cells. T2 B cells differentiate into either follicular (FO) B cells or marginal zone (MZ) B cells depending on signals received through the BCR and other receptors. Once differentiated, they are now considered mature B cells, or naive B cells.

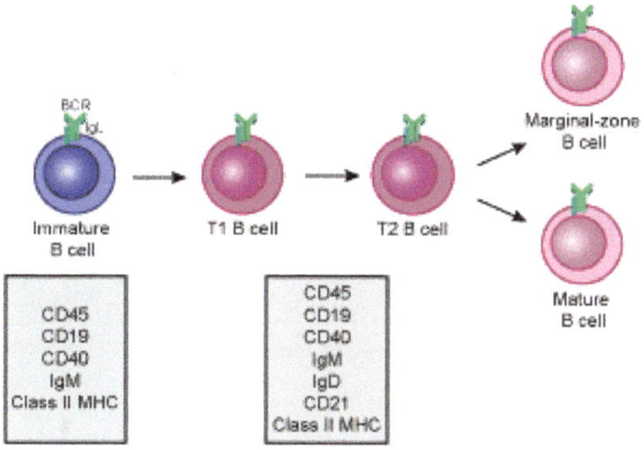

Transitional B cell development: from immature B cell to MZ B cell or mature (FO) B cell

While immature and during the T1 phase, B cells express BCRCR of class IgH, but BCR expression changes to the classes IgM and IgD after transition into the T2 phase and while mature up to activation.

Activation

B cell activation occurs in the secondary lymphoid organs (SLOs), such as the spleen and lymph nodes. After B cells mature in the bone marrow, they migrate through the blood to SLOs, which receive a constant supply of antigen through circulating lymph. At the SLO, B cell activation begins when the B cell binds to an antigen via its BCR. Antigen is presented to lymphocytes by APCs such as macrophages or dendritic cells (DCs), and include proteins, glycoproteins, polysaccharides, whole virus particles, and whole bacterial cells. Of the three B cell subsets, FO B cells preferentially undergo T cell-dependent activation while MZ B cells and B1 B cells preferentially undergo T cell-independent activation.

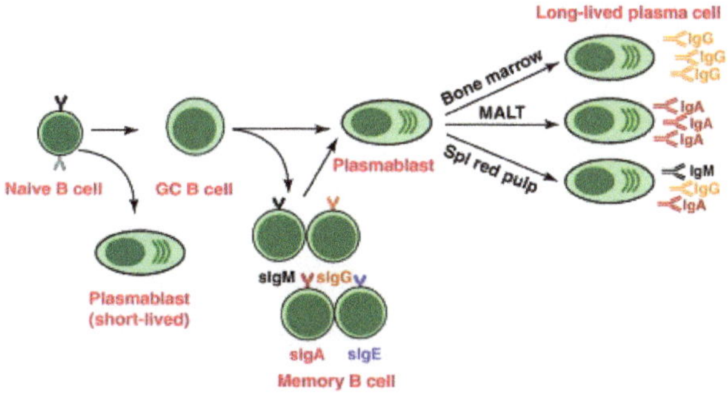

B cell activation: from immature B cell to plasma cell or memory B cell

B cell activation is enhanced through the activity of CD21, a surface receptor in complex with surface proteins CD19 and CD81 (all three are collectively known as the B cell coreceptor complex). When a BCR binds an antigen tagged with a fragment of the C3 complement protein, CD21 binds the C3 fragment, co-ligates with the bound BCR, and signals are transduced through CD19 and CD81 to lower the activation threshold of the cell.

T Cell-dependent Activation

Antigens that activate B cells with the help of T-cell are known as T cell-dependent (TD) antigens and include foreign proteins. They are named as such because they are unable to induce a humoral response in organisms that lack T cells. B cell response to these antigens takes multiple days, though antibodies generated have a higher affinity and are more functionally versatile than those generated from T cell-independent activation.

Once a BCR binds a TD antigen, the antigen is taken up into the B cell through receptor-mediated endocytosis, degraded, and presented to T cells as peptide pieces in complex with MHC-II molecules on the cell membrane. T helper (T_H) cells, typically follicular T helper (T_{FH}) cells, that were activated with the same antigen recognize and bind these MHC-II-peptide complexes through their T cell receptor (TCR). Following TCR-MHC-II-peptide binding, T cells express the surface protein CD40L as well as cytokines such as IL-4 and IL-21. CD40L serves as a necessary co-stimulatory factor for B cell activation by binding the B cell surface receptor CD40, which promotes B cell proliferation, immunoglobulin class switching, and somatic hypermutation as well as sustains T cell growth and differentiation. T cell-derived cytokines bound by B cell cytokine receptors also promote B cell proliferation, immunoglobulin class switching, and somatic hypermutation as well as guide differentiation. After B cells receive these signals, they are considered activated.

Now activated, B cells participate in a two-step differentiation process that yields both short-lived plasmablasts for immediate protection and long-lived plasma cells and memory B cells for persistent protection. The first step, known as the extrafollicular response, occurs outside of lymphoid follicles but still in the SLO. During this step activated B cells proliferate, may undergo immunoglobulin class switching, and differentiate into plasmablasts that produce early, weak antibodies mostly of class IgM. The second step consists of activated B cells entering a lymphoid follicle and forming a germinal center (GC), which is a specialized microenvironment where B cells undergo extensive proliferation, immunoglobulin class switching, and affinity maturation directed by somatic hypermutation. These processes are facilitated by T_{FH} cells within the GC and generate both high-affinity memory B cells and long-lived plasma cells. Resultant plasma cells secrete large amounts of antibody and either stay within the SLO or, more preferentially, migrate to bone marrow.

T Cell-independent Activation

Antigens that activate B cells without T cell help are known as T cell-independent (TI) antigens and include foreign polysaccharides and unmethylated CpG DNA. They are named as such because they are able to induce a humoral response in organisms that lack T cells. B cell response to these antigens is rapid, though antibodies generated tend to have lower affinity and are less functionally versatile than those generated from T cell-dependent activation.

As with TD antigens, B cells activated by TI antigens need additional signals to complete activation, but instead of receiving them from T cells, they are provided either by recognition and binding of a common microbial constituent to toll-like receptors (TLRs) or by extensive crosslinking of BCRs to repeated epitopes on a bacterial cell. B cells activated by TI antigens go on to proliferate outside of lymphoid follicles but still in SLOs (GCs do not form), possibly undergo immunoglobulin class switching, and differentiate into short-lived plasmablasts that produce early, weak antibodies mostly of class IgM, but also some populations of long-lived plasma cells.

Memory B Cell Activation

Memory B cell activation begins with the detection and binding of their target antigen, which is shared by their parent B cell. Some memory B cells can be activated without T cell help, such as certain virus-specific memory B cells, but others need T cell help. Upon antigen binding, the memory B cell takes up the antigen through receptor-mediated endocytosis, degrades it, and presents it to T cells as peptide pieces in complex with MHC-II molecules on the cell membrane. Memory T helper (T_H) cells, typically memory follicular T helper (T_{FH}) cells, that were derived from T cells activated with the same antigen recognize and bind these MHC-II-peptide complexes through their TCR. Following TCR-MHC-II-peptide binding and the relay of other signals from the memory T_{FH} cell, the memory B cell is activated and differentiates either into plasmablasts and plasma cells via an extrafollicular response or enter a germinal center reaction where they generate plasma cells and more memory B cells. It is unclear whether the memory B cells undergo further affinity maturation within these secondary GCs.

B Cell Types

- Plasmablast - A short-lived, proliferating antibody-secreting cell arising from B cell differentiation. Plasmablasts are generated early in an infection and their antibodies tend to have a weaker affinity towards their target antigen compared to plasma cell. Plasmablasts can result from T cell-independent activation of B cells or the extrafollicular response from T cell-dependent activation of B cells.
- Plasma cell - A long-lived, non-proliferating antibody-secreting cell arising from B cell differentiation. There is evidence that B cells first differentiate into

a plasmablast-like cell, then differentiate into a plasma cell. Plasma cells are generated later in an infection and, compared to plasmablasts, have antibodies with a higher affinity towards their target antigen due to affinity maturation in the germinal center (GC) and produce more antibodies. Plasma cells typically result from the germinal center reaction from T cell-dependent activation of B cells, however they can also result from T cell-independent activation of B cells.

- Memory B cell - Dormant B cell arising from B cell differentiation. Their function is to circulate through the body and initiate a stronger, more rapid antibody response (known as the secondary antibody response) if they detect the antigen that had activated their parent B cell (memory B cells and their parent B cells share the same BCR, thus they detect the same antigen). Memory B cells can be generated from T cell-dependent activation through both the extrafollicular response and the germinal center reaction as well as from T cell-independent activation of B1 cells.
- Follicular (FO) B Cell (also known as a B-2 cell) - Most common type of B cell and, when not circulating through the blood, is found mainly in the lymphoid follicles of secondary lymphoid organs (SLOs). They are responsible for generating the majority of high-affinity antibodies during an infection.
- Marginal zone (MZ) B cell - Found mainly in the marginal zone of the spleen and serves as a first line of defense against blood-borne pathogens, as the marginal zone receives large amounts of blood from the general circulation. They can undergo both T cell-independent and T cell-dependent activation, but preferentially undergo T cell-independent activation.
- B-1 cell - Arises from a developmental pathway different from FO B cells and MZ B cells. In mice, they predominantly populate the peritoneal cavity and pleural cavity, generate natural antibodies (antibodies produced without infection), defend against mucosal pathogens, and primarily exhibit T cell-independent activation. A true homologue of mouse B-1 cells has not been discovered in humans, though various cell populations similar to B-1 cells have been described.
- B-2 cell - FO B cells and MZ B cells.
- Regulatory B (Breg) cell - An immunosuppressive B cell type that stops the expansion of pathogenic, pro-inflammatory lymphocytes through the secretion of IL-10, IL-35, and TGF-β. Also, it promotes the generation of regulatory T (Treg) cells by directly interacting with T cells to skew their differentiation towards Tregs. No common Breg cell identity has been described and many Breg cell subsets sharing regulatory functions have been found in both mice and humans. It is currently unknown if Breg cell subsets are developmentally linked and how exactly differentiation into a Breg cell occurs. There is evidence showing that nearly all B cell types can differentiate into a Breg cell through mechanisms involving inflammatory signals and BCR recognition.

B Cell-related Pathology

Autoimmune disease can result from abnormal B cell recognition of self-antigens followed by the production of autoantibodies. Autoimmune diseases where disease activity is correlated with B cell activity include scleroderma, multiple sclerosis, systemic lupus erythematosus, type 1 diabetes, and rheumatoid arthritis.

Malignant transformation of B cells and their precursors can cause a host of cancers, including chronic lymphocytic leukemia (CLL), acute lymphoblastic leukemia (ALL), hairy cell leukemia, follicular lymphoma, non-Hodgkin's lymphoma, and Hodgkin's lymphoma.

Epigenetic

A study that investigated the methylome of B cells along their differentiation cycle, using whole-genome bisulfite sequencing (WGBS), showed that there is a hypomethylation from the earliest stages to the most differentiated stages. The largest methylation difference is between the stages of germinal center B cells and memory B cells. Furthermore, this study showed that there is a similarity between B cell tumors and long-lived B cells in their DNA methylation signatures.

The humoral immunity is the other essential arm of adaptive immune response which is mainly governed by the antibodies. The humoral immune response is important against extracellular microbes, microbial toxins, fungi, and viruses. Any defect in the production of antibody leads to severe complications in immune compromised individuals. Current day vaccine strategies are mostly directed to increase the antibody production against specific pathogens.

Figure: Overview of effector functions of antibody:

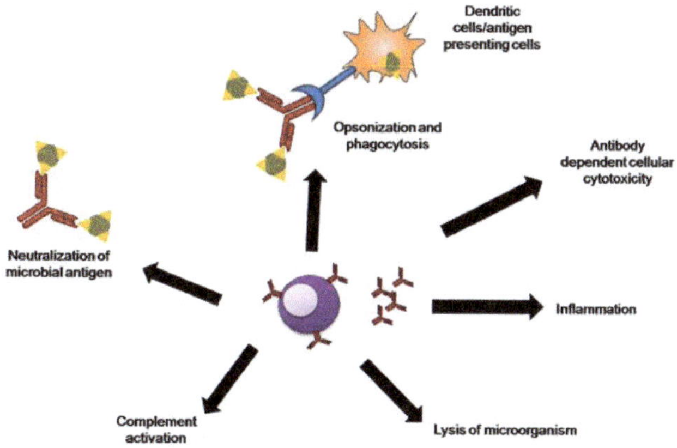

Neutralization of Microorganisms and Their Toxins

Most of the microorganisms attack and enter the host body after binding to a specific cell receptor present over the host cell. The specific structures present over the surface of bacteria, viruses, parasite or fungi are responsible for their attachment to the cell receptors. When the microorganism and its toxin enters or are produced inside the body the host immune system produces the antibody specific to bind their surface molecules. The binding of specific antibodies to these molecules in the microbes and toxin makes it inaccessible to the host cell and hence neutralized. The host cell produces antibodies against the surface glycoprotein hemagglutinin in influenza virus infection in order to inhibit their binding to the sialic acid receptor present on the respiratory epithelium. Similarly, tetanus toxin binds to the cellular receptors over the neurotransmitter junction leading to paralysis and lockjaw condition. The antibody produced in *Clostridium tetani* infection neutralizes the toxins and inhibits its binding to receptors present in the motor end plates. Neutralization of the microbes and their toxins only requires antigen binding region of the antibody, i.e Fab or F $(ab)_2$fragments. Most of the neutralizing antibodies in the blood are of IgG and IgA types in the mucosal surface.

Opsonization and Phagocytosis

Coating of microbes by the IgG type antibody helps in their phagocytosis by macrophages and neutrophils, the phenomenon is called opsonization . The Fc receptor of the IgG containing microbes binds to the neutrophils and participates in their intracellular degradation and killing. In addition to IgG molecules, complement protein C3b also helps in the opsonization and phagocytosis of the microbes by binding to leukocytes. The substance that helps in opsonization and phagocytosis including antibodies and complements are called as opsonins.

Table: Functions of different antibody:

Types	Function
IgG	Neutralization of toxins and microbes. Opsonization of antigens Activation of classical pathway of complement system Antibody dependent cell mediated cytotoxicity Transfer through placenta to neonates Negative feedback to B cell activation
IgA	Neutralization over the mucosal surface Activation of lectin and alternate pathway of complement system
IgM	Activation of classical pathway of complement system Antigen receptor on the naive B cell
IgE	Mast cell degranulation Allergic reaction Immediate type hypersensitivity reaction
IgD	Antigen receptor on the naive B cell

Antibody Dependent Cell-mediated Cytotoxicity

Many subclasses of IgG antibodies bind to infected cells and are recognized by the Fc receptors of NK cell. NK cell contains Fc receptor called FcγRIII (CD16) that binds to the antibody coated infected cells. Many therapeutic monoclonal antibodies against tumor cells are working on the same principle by coating the tumor cells which facilitates their killing by NK cells.

Antibody Dependent Killing of Helminths

Helminths are larger in size and cannot be processed by phagocytic cells of the immune system. Antibodies like IgE, IgG, and IgA coats the surface of helminths which can bind to the Fc receptor present over the eosinophils. Eosinophils contain granules in their cytoplasm which are responsible for the secretion of microbicidal major basic proteins . Binding of the antibody coated helminths to Fc receptor degranulates the eosinophils and secretion of major basic protein which is responsible for their killing. Mast cells also take part in the clearance of helminths from the body. Mast cell releases many cytokines and chemokines which attracts and helps in the degranulation of eosinophils and in turns secretion of major basic protein.

The Complement System

The complement system consists of different serum proteins that works through different pathways and interacts with each other in order to kill the invading microbes. The complement system is activated by the microbial antigen and the antibody produced against them by the host immune system. The proteins of the complement system attaches sequentially over the surface of microbes and help in their lysis. The complement system comprises of classical, alternate, and lectin pathways . The classical pathway is activated by the antibody binding with an antigen, alternate pathway activates in absence of antibody, and lectin pathway activates in response of lectin that binds to mannose. The final step in all these three pathways leads to the formation of membrane attack complex. These complexes are around 100 Å in diameter and forms, a channel that allows the free flow of water and ion into the microbial cells. The movement of water and ions inside the cells increases the osmotic pressure of the cells and its rupture. The pore formed by complement proteins are similar to what we observe in case of NK cells, where instead of water and ions, perforin and granzyme enters and kills the cell.

Function of Complement System

- Promotes phagocytosis of the microbes by opsonization.
- Stimulates inflammation by degranulation of mast cells.
- Lysis of microbes by forming a membrane attack complex.

- Solubilization of those complexes that are unwanted for the body and helps in their clearance.

Figure: Different complement pathways:

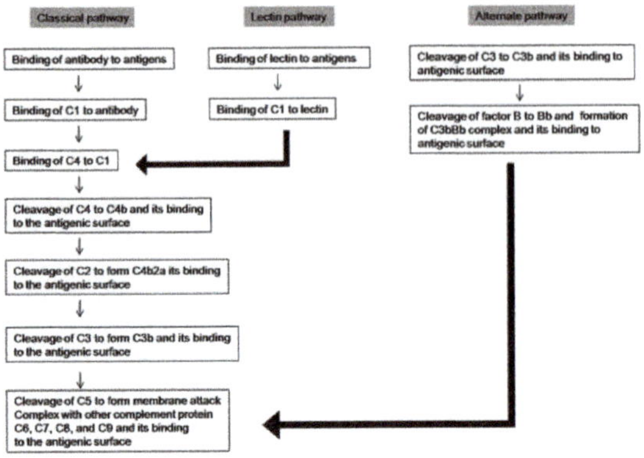

Neonatal Immunity

The body of neonate is sterile and passive transfer of antibody takes place by placenta before birth and through milk immediately after birth. The passive transfer of antibodies to neonates is important in providing immunity during the early phase of life when the immune system is not fully functional. Transfer of antibody through the gut in early life phase is called transcytosis. The maternal IgG is transferred through placenta and IgG and IgA through milk.

Permissions

All chapters in this book are published with permission under the Creative Commons Attribution Share Alike License or equivalent. Every chapter published in this book has been scrutinized by our experts. Their significance has been extensively debated. The topics covered herein carry significant information for a comprehensive understanding. They may even be implemented as practical applications or may be referred to as a beginning point for further studies.

We would like to thank the editorial team for lending their expertise to make the book truly unique. They have played a crucial role in the development of this book. Without their invaluable contributions this book wouldn't have been possible. They have made vital efforts to compile up to date information on the varied aspects of this subject to make this book a valuable addition to the collection of many professionals and students.

This book was conceptualized with the vision of imparting up-to-date and integrated information in this field. To ensure the same, a matchless editorial board was set up. Every individual on the board went through rigorous rounds of assessment to prove their worth. After which they invested a large part of their time researching and compiling the most relevant data for our readers.

The editorial board has been involved in producing this book since its inception. They have spent rigorous hours researching and exploring the diverse topics which have resulted in the successful publishing of this book. They have passed on their knowledge of decades through this book. To expedite this challenging task, the publisher supported the team at every step. A small team of assistant editors was also appointed to further simplify the editing procedure and attain best results for the readers.

Apart from the editorial board, the designing team has also invested a significant amount of their time in understanding the subject and creating the most relevant covers. They scrutinized every image to scout for the most suitable representation of the subject and create an appropriate cover for the book.

The publishing team has been an ardent support to the editorial, designing and production team. Their endless efforts to recruit the best for this project, has resulted in the accomplishment of this book. They are a veteran in the field of academics and their pool of knowledge is as vast as their experience in printing. Their expertise and guidance has proved useful at every step. Their uncompromising quality standards have made this book an exceptional effort. Their encouragement from time to time has been an inspiration for everyone.

The publisher and the editorial board hope that this book will prove to be a valuable piece of knowledge for students, practitioners and scholars across the globe.

Index

T

V